Commen   *our fingertips* from readers

'I enjoye   ...ations to the ...uthors.'

Dr ALISON JONES
Consultant Medical Oncologist
Royal Free Hampstead NHS Trust

'. . . this is a beneficial book for women recently diagnosed with breast cancer and their relatives.'

GERALD GUI
Consultant Breast Surgeon
Royal Marsden Hospital

'. . . packed with good factual information about breast cancer'

VIRGINIA STRAKER
Breast Care Nurse, Winchester

Breast cancer

Answers at your fingertips

Emma Pennery
Val Speechley
Maxine Rosenfield

CLASS PUBLISHING · LONDON

The authors and publisher welcome feedback from the users of this book. Please contact the publisher:

Class Publishing Ltd, Barb House, Barb Mews, London W6 7PA, UK
Telephone: 020 7371 2119
Fax: 020 7371 2878 [International +4420]
email: post@class.co.uk
Website: www.class.co.uk

A CIP catalogue for this book is available from the British Library.

ISBN 978 1 85959 198 7

10 9 8 7 6 5 4 3 2 1

Edited by Caroline Sheldrick

Cartoons by Jane Taylor

Line illustrations by David Woodroffe

Designed and typeset by Martin Bristow

Printed and bound by WS Bookwell, Juva

Contents

Foreword

by **Diana Moran**
The 'Green Goddess'

Oh how I wish this excellent book had been available to me 21 years ago, when I travelled the road of my traumatic breast cancer alone. But it had yet to be written, so I experienced my bumpy, sometimes frightening ride without a lot to read to prepare me for the hazards I encountered around the bends.

Times have changed for the better, and with the help of this book, women, their families and friends – and not forgetting some men – now have at their fingertips first-class information about the disease and ways to combat it. Arming oneself with information is the best way I know to acquire strength. Knowledge can help dispense fear and equip us to cope with the unknown.

The following pages are full of sound knowledge, facts about breast cancer and expert advice. The latest information is given in a straightforward way which creates a calm response to diagnosis and a positive approach to recommended treatments. I like this book for the ease in which I can find concise answers to my questions, clear explanations, diagrams to illustrate the points and practical suggestions.

It is interesting that many of the questions posed are the same ones I wanted answers to all those years ago. Whoever we are, whatever our age, colour, class or creed, we all look for an answer to the question 'why me?' We all experience confusion, anger, distress and fright in varying degrees from the first signs and symptoms through to the diagnosis of breast cancer.

With its up-to-date advice on latest research and treatments, the authors hold our hand and guide us through the breast cancer journey. By explaining how we are all unique and that all cancers are dissimilar they dispel unfounded myths, explain the benefits of complementary therapies and help us understand and come to terms with diagnosis and recommended treatment.

If you are embarking on your journey, or travelling down the road for a second time, my personal tip is to make a list of your concerns and to keep asking questions. Dip in and out of the book, take note of any advice you are given, and if you are unsure of anything or have specific concerns ask your medical team. The cancer support organisations, counsellors and websites, whose details are given in the Appendix, are also excellent sources of information.

It is so important that you digest and think all the information through. You need to be sure before you make any decisions. For you alone must feel confident enough to give your consent before the doctors, or other staff, can proceed with recommended surgery, treatment and care.

As you make your journey you may discover a positive and unexpected benefit from your breast cancer experience. As a survivor I know, because it happened to me. Your view of life may sharpen and life itself may feel richer and more precious from the experience: I don't intend to waste a single day!

With my love and understanding

Diana Moran.

Foreword

by **Professor Ian Smith**
Professor of Cancer Medicine, Royal Marsden NHS Trust

Breast cancer is becoming one of the success stories of modern medicine. More and more women all over the world are developing the disease each year, but more and more are also surviving, and breast cancer mortality has been falling steadily over the past 20 years. This may be partly because it is diagnosed earlier, but it is mainly because of the introduction of adjuvant medical therapy (anti-hormonal therapy, chemotherapy and recently, biological therapy, also called targeted therapy) given immediately after surgery when the disease is still at an early stage and potentially curable. Today the diagnosis and treatment of breast cancer is a team effort with surgeons, physicians, radiation oncologists, pathologists, radiologists and nurses working together as an integrated team.

Breast cancer raises many questions in the minds of patients, their families and friends and indeed in many well women anxious to avoid the disease. This timely book addresses these questions and answers them clearly and sensibly. Time and again as I read the book I heard the voices of my own patients asking the same questions. The different treatment options and their side effects, the difference between stage and grade, the role of dairy foods and diet in general, what to tell the children, and the role of complementary therapies – no important issues are left out.

It is no coincidence that the authors are nurses. In today's modern multi-disciplinary breast clinic, the nurse has a central and crucial role in guiding and supporting patients through complex treatment choices. No one is better placed than the authors to understand the issues, the underlying anxieties and the best way to help. This is a book for everyone whose life has been touched by breast cancer.

Acknowledgements

We would like to thank our reviewers, Alison Jones, Gerald Gui, Sally Shanley and Ginny Straker for their constructive comments, and to Professor Ian Smith and Diana Moran for the Forewords. Tina Glynn and Caroline Hoffman of the Breast Cancer Haven, London made valuable contributions to the complementary therapies chapter, and David Proudfoot helped with compiling the Appendix. Our grateful thanks also go to The Royal Marsden NHS Foundation Trust for permission to reproduce illustrations from their Patient Information Series of booklets, and to Varian Medical Systems.

Introduction

This book provides information about breast cancer, the treatment options available and ways of living with – and after – treatment for breast cancer. It is intended to be used by people who have, or suspect they may have, breast cancer and their friends and relatives. The book mostly comprises questions and answers which are based on the most commonly asked questions about breast cancer, drawn from various sources including the authors' personal experience.

While the book attempts to touch on all aspects of the disease, we are conscious that there are omissions. To include every possible fact or facet would require an encyclopaedia!

Many organisations produce detailed literature and provide information about aspects of breast cancer and its treatment. You will find we often refer to such organisations rather than duplicating information. They may also be able to guide you to other relevant books. The answers we give may not apply to every person with breast cancer. It is essential, if you have breast cancer, to ask questions of doctors, nurses and other healthcare professionals. It is equally important that you gain easy, unprejudiced access to the various voluntary and supportive services. If you do this, you should have a better understanding of this experience and of how to live life with, and after, breast cancer.

The chapters are arranged to answer questions about breast cancer facts, how a breast cancer diagnosis is made, the treatments which may be offered, their possible side effects, complementary therapies which may be used and the ways in which breast cancer can affect your lifestyle.

You may decide to read the book from cover to cover, but it has been written so that you can choose the parts in which you are most interested. For this reason, some of the information is given in more than one chapter, but we think it is better to repeat information wherever it might be needed rather than expect you to keep moving from one place in the book to another. There is a glossary of terms used in the text at the back of the book for quick reference.

We would like to know if there are important questions we have not covered (which we may be able to incorporate in a later edition) and we would also welcome any other comments you may have on this book. Please write to us c/o Class Publishing, Barb House, Barb Mews, London W6 7PA, UK.

1 | What is breast cancer?

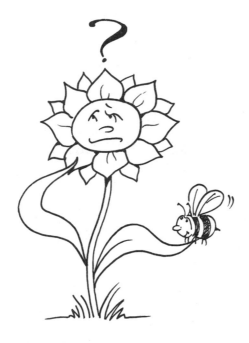

Cancer is a word that is used to describe about 200 different diseases affecting organs or systems of the body. Each type of cancer has its own possible causes, and develops and behaves in its own way. Breast cancer is explained here, with descriptions of the different types and what might cause them to occur.

BREAST CANCER

All cancers are diseases of cells. Cells are the smallest building blocks in our bodies, invisible to the naked eye. Groups of cells form the tissues and organs of the body (such as the breasts, liver or lungs) and each of these has a very specific function.

Cells normally reproduce themselves by dividing in a regular, orderly fashion so that body tissues can grow and repair any damage. If this normal function is disrupted, there may be an uncontrolled growth of cells forming a lump called a tumour. There are two kinds of tumour, benign and malignant, and the malignant ones are called cancer.

Most tumours in the breast are **benign.** This means they remain contained within a localised area, cannot spread and often do not require any treatment as they do not do any harm. An example of a common benign breast tumour is a **fibroadenoma** (an overgrowth of normal tissue that forms a lump). Sometimes an operation is needed to remove a fibroadenoma because it is large or uncomfortable but in most cases such a lump can safely be left alone.

Malignant breast tumours (cancer) can also grow in the breast. These are different to benign tumours because they have developed, or can develop, the ability to spread either to surrounding tissue or elsewhere in the body. This process is called **metastasis.** Breast cancer cells spread elsewhere by breaking off the original breast tumour and travelling in the bloodstream to distant sites in the body where they may form new tumours called **metastases** or **secondaries**. Cancer cells may also be carried away from the breast in the lymphatic system, which normally helps the body to fight infection. This system is made up of **lymph nodes** (glands) and vessels (tubes) linked throughout the body. The lymphatic system drains the fluid **lymph** from different parts of the body and returns it to the bloodstream.

Because breast cancer cells can spread to vital organs (such as the liver or lungs) and affect their normal function, secondary breast cancer anywhere in the body can be a life-threatening disease.

Both women and men can develop breast cancer, although it is very rare in men.

Are there different types of breast cancer?

Yes. Most breast cancers are a type of cancer called **carcinomas**. These arise from the cells lining an organ or system. Within our breasts, there are lobules (where in women milk is made and stored)

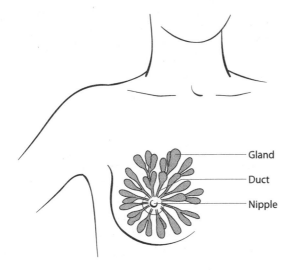

Figure 1 Structure of the breast

and ducts (tubes which carry milk to the nipple). Breast cancers that start in the lobules are called **invasive lobular carcinoma** and breast cancers that start in the ducts are called **invasive ductal carcinoma**.

There is also a very early type of breast cancer called **ductal carcinoma in situ** (DCIS). This is when cancer cells are found in the ducts but have not yet developed the ability to spread. It usually needs to be removed because in some cases the DCIS will go on to become invasive breast cancer and could therefore spread at some point in the future.

There are also other less common types of breast cancer such as inflammatory breast cancer, malignant phyllodes and Paget's disease.

Do all types of breast cancer behave in the same way?

No. Different breast cancers behave in their own way and grow at different rates. Some are more likely to be treated successfully than others. We still don't fully understand why breast cancers can behave differently and why some respond better to treatment than others.

Scientists are, however, beginning to identify and understand various sub-types and this may help predict a person's chances of survival and indicate how best to treat them. Each sub-type of breast cancer is made up of different tissues because of the different proteins inside it. Sub-types identified so far include luminal and basal, but as there are breast cancers that don't yet fit in any sub-type, more research is needed.

Why did my friend's breast cancer come back years after it was treated?

Breast cancers usually take many months or even years to grow to the size they are when they can be diagnosed. During this period there is plenty of time for cells to break off the original tumour and spread to other parts of the body (called **secondary** or **metastatic breast cancer**). At the time of diagnosis, these secondary breast cancers may be too small to be detected. Even if all the original cancer seems to have been removed, or there is no evidence of cancer after treatment, the secondary breast cancers may already be growing at other sites. They may stay 'silent' for months or years, just as the original cancer did, until the cells reach sufficient numbers to cause a new symptom. It only requires one breast cancer cell to be left undetected or untreated for the disease to recur in the future. This is what probably happened in your friend's case.

Secondary breast cancer cells spread to other parts of the body from the first, or primary, tumour in the breast through the lymphatic or blood system. When breast cancer spreads, for example to the bones, it is called **secondary breast cancer in the bone**. This is because the cancer cells in the bone are breast cancer cells.

If breast cancer comes back in either the same breast or near the mastectomy scar, it is called a **local recurrence**. When it spreads to areas around the breast such as the skin, the muscles on the chest wall, the lymph nodes under the sternum (breastbone), between the ribs or the nodes above the clavicle (collarbone) it is called **regional recurrence**.

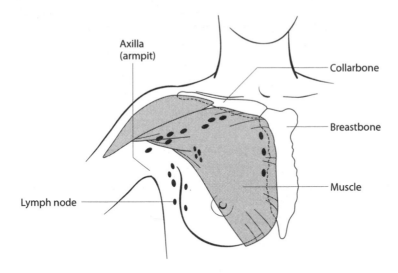

Figure 2 Structure of the breast area

I see a lot about breast cancer in newspapers and magazines now, and more on television. Is breast cancer becoming more common?

Breast cancer is the most common cancer in the UK. How many people get a certain type of cancer each year is called the **incidence** and the incidence of breast cancer is increasing every year. There are several reasons for this. We all live longer nowadays which means there is more time for breast cancer to develop. We are also better at finding breast cancers now, specifically through the national **screening** programme (see Chapter 2). Finally there have been lifestyle changes in the population, in that we eat differently, drink more alcohol and more of us are overweight.

In 2004 over 44,600 cases of breast cancer were diagnosed. More than 44,300 of these were in women, with just 300 cases in men.

Is breast cancer the main cause of death in this country?

Breast cancer is the second biggest cause of death from cancer in women in the UK (lung cancer is the biggest). But overall there are many more deaths in women, and men, caused by cardiovascular disease (heart attacks and strokes).

I am nearly 45. What is my chance of getting breast cancer?

Across your whole lifetime your chance as a woman of getting breast cancer is one in nine, but this is cumulative, meaning that the risk increases as you get older. In younger women, the chances are much less. Up to the age of 30 you have only a one in 1,900 chance of getting breast cancer. Your individual risk of breast cancer can also be affected by the risk factors explained below.

If I do get breast cancer I'll probably die from it, won't I?

No, in fact most people are alive many years after a diagnosis of breast cancer. Survival figures for breast cancer are usually given in terms of five-year, ten-year and twenty-year survival, which is the percentage of people alive that many years after they were first diagnosed and treated. In the UK, 80% are alive at five years after a diagnosis of **primary breast cancer**; at 10 years this is 72% and at 20 years the survival is 64%. Not everyone still alive at these time points will be cured; some may already have had a recurrence of their breast cancer and for some it may return later.

What causes breast cancer?

Every cell in the body contains a set of instructions (its genetic material) which controls the way it grows and behaves. Cancer happens when changes take place in this genetic material so that the cells no longer behave normally and instead grow in an uncontrolled way. There are many reasons why this may happen. In some cancers, the causes are much clearer (there is far more evidence), for example smoking and lung cancer, but with breast cancer a definite cause is harder to pinpoint. This is why health professionals will more commonly talk about **risk factors**, rather than causes. Risk factors are things that affect the chances of breast cancer developing in an individual person, either increasing or decreasing their risk.

What are the main risk factors for breast cancer?

The two biggest things that increase our risk of developing breast cancer are our sex and our age, neither of which we can do anything about. Just being a woman puts people at most risk because nearly all breast cancers occur in women. Getting older also increases the risk because most cases (over 80%) occur in women aged 50 years and over. Breast cancer is much less common in younger women.

In men, where breast cancer is more rare, there are some known risk factors, for example:

- Increasing age (it is more common over 60 years of age);

- Radiation (for example, previous treatment for Hodgkin's disease) but this accounts for a tiny number of cases;

- Obesity (being overweight);

- An inherited faulty gene (affecting less than 10% of breast cancers in women and 15% of all breast cancers in men);

- High oestrogen levels (for example, due to obesity or chronic liver damage);

- Klinefelter's syndrome (an extra female **chromosome**, which is very rare).

I started my periods rather late. Does that make a difference?

There is a slight increase in breast cancer risk the earlier a girl starts her periods and the later a woman begins the menopause. This is because some breast cancers use the female hormone oestrogen to help them grow. There is more of this hormone circulating around the body after puberty and before the menopause.

The average age for starting your periods is around 13 years old but if they start earlier, this increases the amount of time that a woman is exposed to circulating hormones. So, since you started late your risk may be lower than average.

Similarly, most women go through the menopause at 50 or 51 years of age. If this happens later than average, say in their mid- to late fifties, it also slightly increases the risk of breast cancer.

My wife believes that having had children and breastfeeding them protects her from breast cancer. Is she right?

She has the right idea. Having children and having them earlier in life (for example in your twenties) results in a lower risk of developing breast cancer than having children later or not at all, and the risk gets slightly less the more children a woman has.

Breastfeeding also reduces the risk of breast cancer but only by a little and only if done for a year or more – though not necessarily all at once: feeding two children for six months each would still count. Generally the longer a woman breastfeeds the more her risk of breast cancer reduces but it is still a very small reduction overall.

I am having trouble with the menopause and thinking about HRT. But does it cause breast cancer?

Taking HRT (hormone replacement therapy) for less than five years will have a negligible effect on your breast cancer risk. However, if you take it for longer than this your risk may increase. It also increases if it is combination HRT, containing oestrogen and progesterone rather than oestrogen only. This risk falls a few years after the HRT is stopped.

It is a personal decision whether or not to take HRT. It is important to weigh the benefits to you, in reducing difficult menopausal symptoms, with your individual risks. Talk over the pros and cons with a doctor or practice nurse to help you reach an informed decision.

I have heard that taking the contraceptive pill may cause breast cancer, so should I avoid it?

It used to be thought that taking the Pill did slightly increase the risk of breast cancer. Recent studies, however, have found no more women get breast cancer who have taken the Pill than those who have never taken it.

Your choice of contraception has to be a personal matter, and you should talk over the advantages and disadvantages of each method with a doctor or practice nurse. That way you and your partner can make an informed decision.

I have put on quite a lot of weight recently. Do weight and exercise really make a difference to the risk of breast cancer?

Being overweight does increase your risk of breast cancer, particularly after the menopause. It seems the more weight you put on over your lifetime, the higher the risk of breast cancer developing after menopause. There are also many other good reasons for keeping your weight within the normal range for your height, not least that it will reduce your risk of developing heart disease and diabetes.

Taking regular exercise (at least 30 minutes a day, five times a week) also reduces the risk of breast cancer and as with weight gain, this seems even more important in reducing the risk in post-menopausal women.

My partner and I enjoy a few drinks most evenings. Should I worry about alcohol and my risk of breast cancer?

The more a woman drinks the greater the risk of developing breast cancer. The risk increases very slightly with every extra unit of alcohol you drink each day, and more so with regular binge drinking.

This doesn't mean that you should give up alcohol altogether. The golden rule is to drink in moderation. Try to follow guidelines on the recommended safe amounts of alcohol: for women, no more than two units per day (one unit of alcohol is half a pint of beer or cider, one small glass of wine or a single measure of spirits).

We have had quite a lot of cancer in our family. Can you inherit breast cancer?

The vast majority of breast cancers happen by chance because it is a very common disease worldwide. However, in a very small number of cases (less than 10%) it can run in families, when it is called **familial** or **hereditary** breast cancer. Overall, less than one woman in 100 is at high risk of developing inherited breast cancer, which is passed on in a faulty **gene**.

The genes we know most about are called **BRCA1**, **BRCA2** and **TP53**. If the faulty genes are confirmed (or are extremely likely because of the patterns of affected relatives), the problem is hereditary. However, if there are several cases in the family, but no obvious pattern or confirmed gene mutation, we may call it familial.

Not every family member will inherit the faulty gene because we all inherit two copies of each of our genes – one copy from our mother and one copy from our father. If your mother or father carries a faulty gene s/he will also have a normal copy. This means that you have a 50:50 chance of inheriting the faulty copy and a 50:50 chance of inheriting the normal copy. If you inherit the faulty copy you have a 50:50 chance of passing it on to your children. If you don't inherit the faulty gene, you can't pass it on to your children.

We can begin to suspect the possibility of inherited breast cancer if there have been more relatives affected in one family than one would expect (multiple cases). Broadly speaking, people have a higher risk than average of developing breast cancer, which across a lifetime is one in nine, if they have any of the following in their family:

- a female **first-degree relative** (mother, daughter or sister) who developed breast cancer at a young age (under 40);

- two first-degree relatives, or one first-degree and one second-degree male or female relatives (grandparents, grandchildren, uncles, aunts, nieces, nephews) who both developed breast cancer under an average age of 50;

- a first-degree male relative (father, brother or son) who developed breast cancer at any age;

- a first-degree relative who developed breast cancer in both breasts (bilateral breast cancer), particularly if under 50 years of age;

- three first- or second-degree relatives who developed breast cancer at younger than an average age of 60;

- four or more relatives who developed breast cancer at any age.

If you are concerned about familial or hereditary breast cancer, the first step is to talk things over with your G`P. Your doctor should ask about family history and ethnic background. This is because the chances of breast cancer being inherited are higher in some ethnic communities, such as Ashkenazi Jewish people. They will also want to know about any blood relatives who have had breast or related cancers (such as ovarian cancer that can be caused by the same faulty gene) and their age when the cancer developed. They then estimate the risk, and if it is considered moderate or high you will be referred for more specialist advice, for example to a cancer genetics centre. Here, the staff will offer to take a detailed family tree to work out the risk.

People at higher risk will be offered genetic counselling to help them understand their risk and all the implications to them and other family members (see below).

Can I be tested for a faulty gene?

Yes, but *only* those in a high-risk group will be offered genetic testing. There are several steps to the testing process. First, a blood sample is taken, ideally from a living relative with breast cancer so that the exact fault on the gene can be identified. This can take many weeks, or even months. If no faulty gene is found, you will not need to be tested. This doesn't mean that a fault does not exist, as it could be on a part of a gene that cannot be detected by current technology.

If a faulty gene is found, the test can then be offered to other relatives who have not yet had breast cancer. This is because the genetics experts will know exactly what gene fault to look for in the other family members. An unaffected relative with the same gene fault is at high risk of developing breast cancer. Family members without the gene fault and who are not affected by breast cancer will be at no more risk than anyone else in the population, and neither will their children.

Remember, though, that even a person at high risk will not necessarily develop breast cancer.

Do all women or men who carry a faulty gene get breast cancer?

No, carrying a faulty BRCA 1 or BRCA 2 gene gives, at most, up to around an 80% chance of developing breast cancer across the lifetime, so it is never certain.

With BRCA1 the lifetime risk of breast cancer for women by age 70 is up to 80% (the risk declines significantly with age) and there is a 12–60% lifetime risk of ovarian cancer.

With BRCA2 the lifetime risk of breast cancer for women by age 70 is up to 80% but the risk does not decline significantly with age and there is a 10–27% lifetime risk of ovarian cancer.

With BRCA2 there is also a greater risk for men to be affected. Breast cancer in men is much rarer but when it does develop about 15% will be hereditary (compared to just 5% in women). If men do inherit a faulty gene their lifetime risk of developing breast cancer is under 10% (compared to 40–80% in women with a faulty gene).

I have been told my risk is higher than average. What are my options?

The action most guaranteed to drastically reduce risk is a **bilateral risk-reducing mastectomy** (having both breasts removed). This is a serious undertaking, and any woman considering it must usually have a faulty gene confirmed or at least be at high risk (usually three times the risk in the general population). Counselling and information would be offered to help you decide whether to go ahead with this operation.

Alternatively, women at high risk can have screening by mammogram (breast X-ray) or a magnetic imaging scan (MRI) regularly. This is usually annually up to the age of 50; then they join the national breast screening programme, but they will continue to be screened each year. Men, even those at high risk, are not routinely offered screening but it is available.

There are also trials offering hormone therapies such as tamoxifen and anastrozole (Arimidex®) to women at high risk (see Chapter 3). Women taking these as a treatment for breast cancer have far fewer new primary breast cancers in the other breast. This suggests these drugs can reduce the chances of breast cancer occurring and so might be useful for women with an increased likelihood of developing the disease. However, they also cause side effects so once again you need to discuss this with the professionals so you can make an informed decision.

Will changing my diet reduce my risk of getting breast cancer?

It is not possible to give a simple answer, as some changes might make a small difference to breast cancer risk, while others will not affect it at all. Studies on diet and risk rely on people accurately recording what they have eaten, so it is hard to determine what exactly in the diet affects risk.

There is, however, convincing evidence that breast cancer risk is slightly increased by:

- a high total dietary fat intake, especially saturated fat (found in meat and dairy products);

- high consumption of red meat (only in older women and those who eat red meat at least once every day).

There is no convincing evidence that eating too many dairy products or white meat or too little fruit, vegetables, fibre and **phyto-oestrogens** (plant based oestrogens such as soya) will increase breast cancer risk. But there is also no evidence to the contrary.

However, eating a well-balanced, healthy diet is recommended to reduce the risk of other illnesses, such as heart disease and diabetes, and to help keep your weight within normal limits (for your height).

There is a lot written about 'super foods'. Is there anything I should eat?

There is no one definition of a 'super food' but generally they refer to foods that are rich in vitamins, antioxidants and **omega-3** oils.

Antioxidants protect our bodies against free radicals, which play a role in ageing and tissue damage that might lead to cancer. They are found mainly in fruit and vegetables. However, whilst fruit and vegetables are important for a healthy diet and have potential anti-cancer properties, there is no evidence that they offer any protection against breast cancer.

Omega-3 oils are part of a healthy diet and help reduce the risk of heart disease. They are found mainly in oily fish and we should eat one or two portions of oily fish a week. Vegetarian sources include linseed and hemp seed. However, as with antioxidants, there is no evidence that they offer any protection against breast cancer.

Does soy help protect against breast cancer?

The number of women getting breast cancer in Asia and Japan is lower than in the Western world and a lot of people claim this is because these women eat more soy. Soy is a phyto-oestrogen (a natural, plant-based oestrogen) and it is thought that phyto-oestrogens contain anti-cancer properties. However, there is no evidence that soy has any effect on breast cancer risk.

Should I only eat organic food because additives cause breast cancer?

Many people believe that breast cancer is linked to additives in our food. But studies have failed to find any link, and no studies have been done which compare organic and non-organic foods to see their effects on breast cancer development.

The safety of food additives and food colourings is governed by the European Food Safety Authority which checks the safety of food additives and makes recommendations about safe quantities and types of additives.

My husband thinks I should take lots of vitamins to protect myself against breast cancer. Will they help?

The only vitamin for which there is some, although not conclusive, evidence is vitamin D. Making sure you have enough vitamin D will very slightly decrease your chances of getting breast cancer. You can get this from sunlight exposure (just a few minutes a day) and foods such as oily fish, eggs and cereals.

Other vitamins are unlikely to have any effect on breast cancer risk. If you eat a well-balanced, healthy diet you should get enough vitamins naturally and not need to take supplements.

Does smoking cause breast cancer? I am thinking of giving up.

We would advise you to give up anyway. Researchers have not agreed about this because some studies have found a slight increase in breast cancer risk among smokers, while others have not. It seems from some studies that any risk might be increased in women who start smoking during their teens. Although we cannot be certain about smoking and breast cancer risk, there is no doubt that smoking is a major cause of lung cancer and heart disease, as well as increasing the risk of cancer of the larynx (voice box) and oesophagus (gullet). Everyone is strongly advised not to smoke but, if you do, seek help to give up.

I have read that underarm deodorants cause breast cancer. Is this true?

Probably not, because there is no convincing evidence to support this – and lots of logical reasons why it is unlikely. Stories have claimed that anti-perspirants and deodorants stop the body from getting rid of toxins (poisons) in sweat and that these toxins could cause breast cancer. But the liver is the main organ used in removing unwanted toxins from the body, whereas the main reason for sweating is to cool the body down. Also, if this were true, we would expect to see more cases of cancer in both breasts, because people use deodorants under both arms, and more breast cancer in men.

I heard a rumour that wearing an underwired bra can mean you will get breast cancer. Should I stop wearing one?

There is no convincing evidence to support this theory and you can safely choose to wear any style of bra – just make sure it fits you well, so that your breasts feel comfortable. A poorly fitting bra can be the cause of breast pain; it's a good idea to be measured once a year.

I carry heavy boxes at work and am always accidentally knocking myself. Will bumps and bruises make me more likely to get breast cancer?

There is no reason to think that this sort of injury will lead to cancer. However, you might want to talk to your line manager about health and safety at work!

I was thinking about having breast implants to make me bigger but then heard that they will increase my risk of breast cancer. Will they?

Breast implants do not affect the risk of cancer developing. However, they can occasionally make it harder for the breasts to be looked at properly on a mammogram (breast X-ray). This can be solved by taking the mammogram pictures from a different angle.

You hear that having an abortion makes breast cancer more likely. Is this true?

There was a study some years ago which seemed to indicate this but more recent studies have shown that having an abortion does not in any way affect the risk of breast cancer.

How do I know if I am at more risk of breast cancer because of where I work?

It is quite normal to worry about whether environmental factors, such as where you work, will affect your chances of getting breast cancer. There has been a lot of research into links between breast cancer and chemicals in our environment such as **pesticides** and **parabens**. However, it is hard to isolate individual chemicals rather than any other factor as the cause of any harmful changes. There is no convincing evidence at present to support this theory and more research is needed.

You should, of course, wear all the recommended protective clothing offered to you at work and follow all the procedures laid down by your employer. If you want to discuss this further, talk to the occupational health department, works doctor, safety representative or your employer. If you're not happy with the answers you get you can contact your local office of the **Health and Safety Executive**, which will be listed in the phone book.

Can you catch breast cancer from someone else?

No. Breast cancer is definitely not infectious or contagious like flu or measles.

I have heard that you can develop breast cancer a few months after a really stressful time. Is this true?

If it were true, it would be hard to prove. We all deal with stress in our own way, and it is very difficult to measure. What one person finds stressful may be exhilarating for someone else. Currently, there is no concrete evidence that stress plays any direct part in the development of breast cancer, but nor is there absolute evidence that it does not. Common sense and experience suggest that we find it hard to deal with all kinds of challenges when we are low. We can be sure that stress which leads us to eat badly, for example too much fat, or drink too much alcohol for any length of time, may influence our breast cancer risk.

2 | Symptoms, screening and investigations

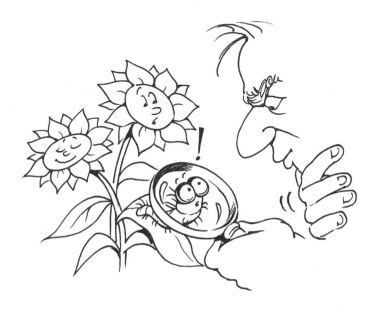

BREAST AWARENESS

The Department of Health (DH) recommends that instead of examining your breasts every month, you should become **breast aware**. Being breast aware means getting to know what is normal for your breasts and knowing what changes to look out for, because this means you will be more likely to notice anything unusual more quickly. Generally the sooner breast cancer is diagnosed and treated, the better the **prognosis** (outcome). So to help people report symptoms quickly, the DH suggests using the following five-point code.

① **Know what is normal for you** Everyone's breasts are a different shape and size, and some people naturally have one breast bigger than the other, so try to become familiar with your normal shape. Remember this will change as we get older, have children and go through the menopause.

② **Know what changes to look and feel for** Most people know that lumps are a possible symptom of breast cancer, but there are other changes that you should report to your doctor without delay (see question below).

③ **Look and feel** Get in to the habit of looking at and feeling your breasts from time to time. Look at your breasts in the mirror and feel them, perhaps when you are in the shower, putting on body lotion or just getting dressed or undressed.

④ **Report any changes to your GP without delay** Your doctor can then reassure you or send you to a breast clinic for more detailed investigations. It is reassuring to know that more than 90% of people referred to a hospital with breast symptoms do *not* have cancer.

⑤ **Attend routine breast screening if you are 50 years of age or over** (see **Screening** below).

The rest of this chapter covers the signs and symptoms of breast cancer, gives details about the NHS Breast Screening Programme and describes some of the more common tests used to confirm or to exclude a diagnosis of breast cancer.

SIGNS AND SYMPTOMS

What symptoms of breast cancer should I look out for?

If you have any of the symptoms listed below, tell your GP about them as soon as possible. If you put off going, you will only worry about it. The chances are there is nothing wrong, but if there is a problem you need to find out quickly. In the less likely event it is breast cancer, the sooner it can be treated the better.

The following are examples of the types of changes which you should report to your GP without delay:

- a change in the size or shape of the breasts – maybe one has got larger or smaller or one seems to be 'pulling' in a different direction;

- changes to the nipple – maybe one is inverted (pulling inwards) or has a rash around it, or there is a discharge leaking from the nipple which might show as a stain in your bra;

- swelling in the armpit area;

- a thickening or lump in the breast that feels different from your usual breast tissue;

- a puckering or dimpling appearance on the skin surface;

- unresolved pain in one part of the breast (rather than all over).

Also, if you have a friend or relative who is worried about any of these things, encourage them to go to the doctor.

I don't like to bother the doctor with something so trivial. They will think I'm just being silly, won't they?

If you notice a breast change that worries you, it is not trivial. The DH recommends that you report breast symptoms without delay. Most doctors are very sympathetic and will listen to what you say, examine you and either set your mind at rest immediately or refer you to a breast clinic for more detailed tests, usually within two weeks. Your doctor has national guidelines about who to refer to a specialist based on their age and the symptoms they have. All people referred urgently (because the GP believes there is a higher chance of it being breast cancer) are seen at the hospital within 10 working days or two calendar weeks (this is called the 'two-week rule'). People referred non-urgently may have to wait longer to be seen but it is still important to have any symptoms checked out just in case.

> *My friend had breast cancer last year. Since then I keep imagining I've got breast cancer every time I get an ache in my breast. Have I got a cancer phobia?*

One of the most common fears people have whenever they notice something unusual in the breast is that they have cancer. This doesn't mean you've got an irrational fear about cancer. Most of us worry about getting ill and are scared of changes we can't explain. Go and talk to your practice nurse or GP. If you don't have any symptoms but are still worried, you may be able to talk with a counsellor, who will help you talk about your fears. Remember to keep being breast aware.

You might also find it helpful to speak to an anonymous person, maybe from a cancer support organisation (see Appendix).

SCREENING

> *My mother had a letter from the doctor which mentioned the NHS Breast Screening Programme. Does that mean she could have cancer?*

No it doesn't. It is a free check-up offered to women over 50 every three years. The NHS Breast Screening Programme was set up as a way of detecting breast cancer at a very early stage because the sooner it is diagnosed the more likely treatment will be successful. Research shows that breast screening saves around 1400 lives every year in England and, for example, that of every 500 women screened, one life will be saved.

Your mother has been invited for breast screening, which involves having a **mammogram** (a breast X-ray) which can detect abnormal changes in the breast that are too small to be felt by the hand. When you have a mammogram you need to undress to the waist and stand in front of an X-ray machine. Each breast is X-rayed in turn by placing it between two X-ray plates. Two views of each breast are taken, one from above and one from the side (diagonally across the breast). Some people find mammograms uncomfortable or even painful but this should pass quickly as soon as the X-ray plates are removed.

The NHS Breast Screening Programme currently offers a free mammogram every three years to all women in the UK aged 50 years and over. Screening services are all staffed entirely by women.

I am 44 now so why don't I get called for breast screening?

Breast cancer is much more common in women over the age of 49 years. In fact 80% of breast cancers occur in older women so it makes sense to screen this age group as this is where most breast cancers will be found. Mammograms are actually less effective in pre-menopausal women under the age of 50. This is because breast tissue is more dense in younger women which makes it more difficult to

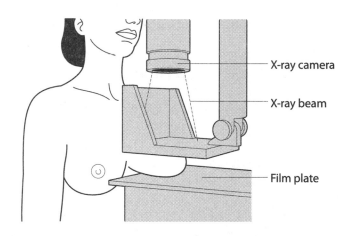

X-ray camera

X-ray beam

Film plate

Figure 3 Having a mammogram

clearly see any abnormal areas. After the menopause breast tissue contains more fatty tissue which is clearer on a mammogram.

Younger women who are not eligible for routine screening but who have symptoms can still be referred to a hospital for tests and these might include a mammogram or an **ultrasound scan** (see question on making a diagnosis, below).

If I'm the right age for screening, will I be called to have a mammogram?

Women aged between 50 and 70 years, identified via GP records, are routinely invited for breast screening. Therefore if you are not registered with an NHS GP you will *not* receive an invitation. You may not receive your invitation as soon as you reach 50 years because people from different GP practices are invited in turn, but you will receive it before your 53rd birthday. Depending on where you live, you will go to a special screening unit, a hospital or a mobile unit (for example in a shopping centre) for your mammogram.

After the age of 70, you are still eligible for free mammograms every three years but you will need to ask for it and make an appointment: you will not receive an automatic invitation after this time. The government has said that screening ages will be extended in the future, to women aged 47–73 years.

How do I find out if my X-ray is normal?

The results of your mammogram will be sent to you and your GP within two weeks.

If I'm called back for a repeat mammogram, does it mean I've got breast cancer?

Only about 5% of women are recalled and of these only around one in eight will be found to have cancer. Most abnormalities seen on a mammogram are benign (or non-cancerous) lumps, such as cysts (fluid-filled lumps). Sometimes a repeat X-ray is needed because there was a technical problem and the picture is not clear. It is important that you attend your second appointment so this can be checked. If further investigations (such as a clinical examination, ultrasound scan or more mammograms at different angles) are necessary these will be carried out as soon as possible.

If my GP or screening doctor sends me to the hospital breast clinic, how will they tell if I have breast cancer?

At the hospital breast clinic you will usually have a combination of tests known as 'triple assessment'.

1. They will take your medical history and examine the breasts, axillae (armpits) and collarbone area.

2. They will do a mammogram and/or an **ultrasound scan** to 'look' inside the breast. Ultrasound scans use sound waves to build up pictures of the inside of the breast. You will need to lie down whilst gel is spread on the breast and a **probe** is passed over the surface of your skin. It is painless and takes a few minutes to do. Ultrasound scans can be useful in younger women, whose breasts are too dense for a clear mammogram and to identify certain types of lumps, such as cysts.

3. If necessary, they will remove some cells or tissue for analysis, either by **fine needle aspiration cytology** (FNAC) which uses a needle to draw off some cells for laboratory analysis, or by **core biopsy** that uses a bigger needle to take out a sliver (small piece) of tissue under a local anaesthetic, which numbs the area.

Some hospitals can give you most of your results on the same day, but others will call you back for them between one and two weeks later. The core biopsy result will take five to seven days.

What happens if the hospital says I have breast cancer?

If the tests show you have breast cancer, your case will then be discussed by the breast unit team. They will be a team made up of breast surgeons, **oncologists** (cancer drug specialists and radio-therapists), **radiologists** (X-ray specialists), **pathologists** (tissue specialists), breast care nurses and others. Together they form a **multi-disciplinary team** (MDT), and they can determine the best course of treatment for you. Possible treatments will then be discussed with you at another appointment. You should meet a breast care nurse at this time. She will be there to give you emotional support and to help answer your questions.

You may need some other investigations (see the next question). The important thing is that you should understand what a test involves and why it is being done. If you don't understand, or you don't remember what you were told the first time, ask again.

Why might I have blood tests?

Blood samples may be taken to assess your general health and how well certain organs in your body, such as liver or kidneys, are functioning. Blood tests are not used to detect the breast cancer itself, and are most commonly done before an operation or before chemotherapy (drug treatment).

SCANS AND TESTS

I am booked in for an MRI scan. What does that involve?

An MRI scan uses a magnetic field to build up extremely detailed pictures of the body. The full name for this investigation is **magnetic resonance imaging**. Computers and radio waves are also used but no radioactive substances. There is usually no special preparation. Not everyone can have this type of scan, for example it isn't suitable for people who have metal in their body such as a heart pacemaker. You cannot take things like keys and watches into the scanning room. Before you come for the scan you may be asked to wear clothes which don't have zips or other metal fastenings, or you might be asked to change into a gown when you arrive.

The scan is not harmful or painful but you will have to lie still for about an hour, usually face down on your tummy, which may be uncomfortable. The table you lie on moves into the scanning machine and so you may feel closed in temporarily. The scanner can be quite noisy at first, but this reduces to tapping sounds later. You may also have an injection of 'contrast' (dye) into a vein in your arm or hand. You should feel no effects from this. The purpose of the contrast is to provide clearer images of certain organs.

Does everyone with breast cancer have an MRI scan?

No, in fact MRI scans are not commonly used in the UK for people with breast cancer. They are not a standard part of triple assessment (see above). Possible reasons for having an MRI scan are:

- to find out more about something abnormal seen on a mammogram;

- to help identify breast cancer in women who have especially dense breast tissue (which can make mammograms hard to read);

- to screen those people at high risk because of a significant family history;

- to assist in screening for cancer in women who have implants or scar tissue from previous surgery, as these might affect the accuracy of a mammogram;

- to determine the integrity of breast implants (looking for ruptures or movement);

- to distinguish between scar tissue and recurrent breast cancer where the difference between the two is unclear.

Will I need a CT scan, and are they like MRI scans?

CT scans (computerised axial tomography) are not usually needed to diagnose anything in breast tissue, but they can be used to look at other parts of the body (such as the lungs or abdomen) if you have any symptoms that might indicate the breast cancer has spread elsewhere in the body.

The CT scanner is a complicated X-ray machine that uses a computer to produce pictures which resemble 'slices' through different parts of your body. You will be asked not to eat or drink for at least a couple of hours before the scan. A CT scan is not harmful or painful but you will have to lie still for up to an hour. The table you lie on can be hard so this may be uncomfortable. The table moves through the X-ray part of the machine as you are being scanned and comes out the other side. So you may feel closed in temporarily. As with an MRI scan, you may have an injection of 'contrast' (dye) into a vein in your arm or hand in order to provide clearer images. Again, you should feel no effects from this.

Why is my friend having a bone scan?

As with MRI and CT scans, bone scans are not routinely done to diagnose breast cancer but can be used either to rule out or confirm a suspicion of breast cancer spreading to the bones, as this is one of the most common places that breast cancer can spread to. Your friend is being checked to see if her cancer has spread this way.

A bone scan is also called an **isotope bone scan**. A small amount of a radioactive substance is injected into a vein, and then there is a wait of two to three hours to allow this to circulate around the skeleton before the scan. Abnormal bone absorbs more radioactivity than normal bone, so the radioactive substance is more visible at sites of abnormal activity (referred to as 'hot spots'). The hot spots could also be caused by arthritis, previous fractures, and so on.

You can go home as soon as the scan has been done, and it is quite safe to have normal contact with people, including children, afterwards.

Why do people with the same diagnosis all have different tests?

Each person is different and will only need the tests that give the medical team the information they need. Don't be alarmed if you have some tests and not others, or if you have an investigation that someone else is not having. The doctors may not need certain scans, for example, to confirm a diagnosis of breast cancer or to help plan treatment.

How long do all these tests take?

The time you may be at the hospital for tests varies. A mammogram or blood test may be over in minutes and a scan may take an hour or more. Occasionally, the preparation for an investigation may take longer than the procedure itself, or you may have to attend more than once during a day – such as for a bone scan. Always ask for details of tests, including the time they take or the time you have to wait. You may wish to take a friend with you, or a book or magazine to read to help pass the time.

How long does it take to get the results of all these tests?

Some test results can be available almost immediately, for example a simple blood test or a routine chest X-ray. But very often the results take days or a couple of weeks to reach your doctor. In the case of a scan, the technician can identify the parts of your body but the pictures produced must be carefully interpreted by a radiologist (a specialist doctor) who will write a report and send it to your doctor. This may take a few days.

Everyone says the waiting is the worst. Is there anything I can do?

Many people find this time the most difficult. It's obviously a time of uncertainty and fear. You may find it helps to talk to your specialist doctors or breast care nurses or to your family doctor. It's also going to be an anxious time for your family. It may help to discuss your fears and concerns with those close to you.

There are also organisations that can provide a listening ear, emotional support and additional information. It may help to talk to people who don't know you, such as a counsellor or someone on a telephone helpline, or to a person who has been through a similar experience. Organisations which offer such help are listed in the Appendix.

What happens when the test results are ready?

When your specialist team has all the results of your tests, they will be able to advise you about what treatments are available, what alternatives exist and what your best course of action might be. It is important that you understand what is said, what is being offered and that you ask all the questions you want.

It can be really helpful to take a friend or relative with you when you go to see your doctor. Make notes and if you want time to think about what has been said, don't be afraid to ask for it. It's not uncommon to have difficulty taking in all the information immediately, so don't feel stupid if you ask about things more than once.

What treatment will I have?

Your treatment will be planned individually for you, and will depend on many factors, including the type of breast cancer, its size, 'grade' and characteristics and your age. Don't be concerned if you speak to people who are having similar, but different, treatments.

Always ask your doctor or breast care nurse about your individual treatment as they will be able to explain exactly what is planned and why. Ideally, you should be given a written copy of your individual treatment plan, although this may change slightly as time goes on. It can take a little time for treatment to be organised, depending on what treatment you are having first. More information about treatment for breast cancer is in Chapter 3.

3 | Treatment and care

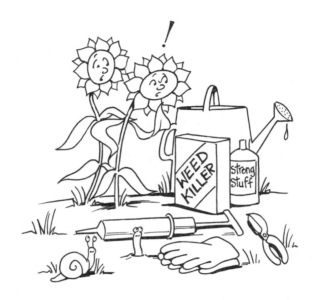

When your specialist team have all the results of your tests and investigations, they will be able to advise you about what sort of treatment you should have. There are five main types of treatment for breast cancer:

- surgery;
- chemotherapy;
- radiotherapy;
- hormone therapy;
- targeted therapy.

Occasionally only one of these is recommended but usually someone will be advised to have a combination of at least two, and often more, types of treatment.

Take every opportunity to discuss your planned treatment and ask questions about it before you make any decisions. Be sure that you understand what the treatment involves before you agree to it. You will need to consent (agree) to any treatment before it starts, and of course you can also refuse treatment if you wish. Your doctors and your breast care nurse will explain what the different treatments involve. They are also there to listen to you and to answer your questions.

Why me? What caused my breast cancer?

Probably everyone who develops cancer asks these questions. Many people ask them when they first hear that they have breast cancer (or suspect they have it), and may ask them repeatedly during any treatment and beyond. One of the hardest things for anyone else to do is to provide an answer, because there isn't one, single explanation. Why you have breast cancer or why it has happened at this point in your life is unlikely to be known. This is little comfort at a time when you are likely to be feeling many mixed emotions. And the last thing you are likely to find helpful is to be told 'not to worry' or to 'put on a brave face' or to feel you have to keep your own feelings inside you to 'protect' others.

Can breast cancer be cured?

Yes, most people treated for breast cancer don't develop recurrent or secondary breast cancer and will live the rest of their lives with no further breast cancer. Unfortunately, not everyone is cured and some people will develop secondary breast cancer which can still be controlled with treatments (sometimes for years) but which cannot be cured.

No doctor or nurse can guarantee anyone a cure but the type of cancer and its characteristics will help them make broad estimates.

How will my specialist team know what treatments might work for me?

They will use the accumulation of many years' experience, and the results of thousands of documented research cases. They will decide which treatments will suit you by taking several factors about your particular type of breast cancer into account. These are some of the factors.

- **The size of the tumour** A large tumour relative to the size of the breast is more likely to require removal of the whole breast (mastectomy).

- **The pattern of the cancer within the breast** If it is in several areas you are more likely to be advised to have the whole breast removed (mastectomy) than if it is confined to one area.

- **How much the cancer cells resemble normal breast tissue** This is called the **grade**.

- **Whether any cancer cells have spread to the lymph glands in the axilla (armpit)** Fluid from the breast drains into the lymph glands in the **axilla** and cancer cells can travel in this fluid.

- **Whether the breast cancer has been stimulated to grow by hormones** This is called **oestrogen** and/or **progesterone positive breast cancer**.

- **Whether the breast cancer has been stimulated to grow by having too much of the protein HER-2** This is called **HER-2 positive breast cancer**, and only occurs in 20% of all invasive breast cancers.

I have been told I have grade 3 breast cancer. What does this mean?

Breast cancers are graded according to how they look under a microscope and how closely they resemble normal breast cells.

The amount of resemblance is called **differentiation**. The less 'differentiated' the cells are, which means they look least like normal breast cells, the faster the cancer cells are growing. There are three grades. Grade 1 is known as low grade; the cancer cells look most like normal breast tissue cells and are said to be 'well differentiated' and grow slower. Grade 3 is known as high grade; the cancer cells have undergone more change and look very different to normal breast cells; they are said to be 'less differentiated' and grow faster.

I have stage II breast cancer. What does that mean?

When people talk about the **stage** of breast cancer, they mean the size of the cancer and its extent – whether it has reached the lymph nodes and whether it has spread elsewhere in the body. In breast cancer there are four main stages.

- Stage I breast cancer is less than 2 cm across and has not spread either to the lymph nodes or elsewhere.

- Stage II breast cancer is between 2 and 5 cm and may have involved the lymph nodes but has not spread to any other parts of the body.

- Stage III breast cancer is larger than 5 cm, may have involved the lymph nodes, the chest muscles or the skin over the breast.

- Stage IV refers to a cancer of any size that has spread to other parts of the body.

I have grade 2, stage I breast cancer. What does that really mean?

A grade 2 cancer means that the cells are 'moderately differentiated' (see question above), look less like normal breast cells and grow slightly faster than normal cells. Stage I means that the cancer is less than 2 cm across and no cancer cells were found in any lymph nodes or anywhere else in your body. Your doctor will use this information to decide on the best treatment to offer you.

SURGERY

Most breast cancers are treated with an operation, aren't they?

Most people with breast cancer will be offered surgery as the first treatment. The aim is to remove the cancer completely from the breast. Broadly speaking, there are two main types of breast cancer operations, **breast conserving surgery** and **mastectomy**. With breast conserving surgery the cancer and a small area of tissue around it (called a margin) is removed. Depending on where the cancer is, and how big it is, this might mean a lumpectomy or the removal of a wider portion of tissue (called a **wide local excision**) where up to a quarter of the breast may be removed.

A mastectomy means all the breast is removed including the nipple.

I have breast cancer and my surgeon says I don't need to have my breast removed; but surely mastectomy is always safer, isn't it?

Not necessarily. Research has shown that people who had operations that conserved the breast and then a course of radiotherapy did just as well as those having a mastectomy. Nowadays, more than half of primary breast cancers are treated with breast conserving surgery and surgeons will try to preserve the breast if at all possible. (A primary breast cancer is one that has started in the breast and is not thought to have spread anywhere else in the body.) There are a few reasons why a mastectomy might be recommended, for example if the cancer is very large in relation to the size of the breast, or if there is more than one area of cancer in your breast. Your surgeon and breast care nurse will explain which type of operation is likely to be best for you and why.

Why do I need to have my lymph nodes removed?

Generally, everyone having breast conserving surgery or mastectomy will have some or all of their lymph nodes in the

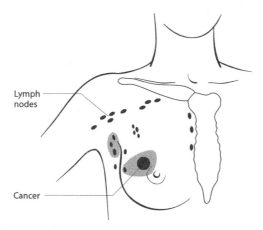

Lymph nodes

Cancer

Figure 4 Tissue removed in a wide local excision (breast conserving surgery)

axilla (armpit) removed. This is called an **axillary dissection**.

Breast cancer can spread to the lymph nodes (see Figure 2, p. 5) and then from there into the rest of the body through the lymphatic system. It is important to remove the nodes to try to prevent further spread but also to help plan what treatment is best for you. If the lymph nodes contain breast cancer cells, you are more likely to have **chemotherapy**, which treats the whole body, because there is a risk that the cancer has spread to other parts of the body. We all have a different number of lymph nodes in the armpit and how many are removed depends on your surgeon as well as on your cancer; some surgeons remove more than others. Most people having an axillary dissection will have between two and twenty removed.

An increasingly common technique used before your operation is called **sentinel lymph node biopsy**. This is a way of checking the lymph nodes to see if the breast cancer has reached them. In this test, a doctor injects a small amount of radioactive material and some blue dye into the breast, some hours before the operation. The nodes that are radioactive, blue or both are called the **sentinel nodes**, and only these (between one and four nodes) are removed during surgery for

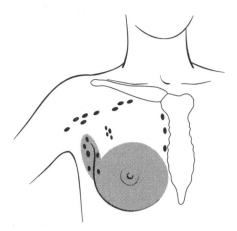

Figure 5 Tissue removed in a mastectomy

testing. If they are free from cancer cells, the other nodes are assumed to be clear as well, and will not be removed unnecessarily. However, if there are cancer cells in the sentinel nodes, then more nodes will need to be removed, usually at a second operation. Sentinel node biopsy should be offered to all people with invasive breast cancer, unless it is already known from a biopsy that the lymph nodes are affected by disease.

If breast cancer has spread to the nodes, it is called **lymph node positive** and if it hasn't, it is called **lymph node negative**.

Can having my lymph nodes removed do me any harm?

People who have surgery to the lymph nodes in the axilla are at risk of developing lymphoedema on that side. **Lymphoedema** is swelling caused by a build-up of lymph fluid in the tissues. It can happen within weeks, months or even years of the surgery, and can affect the whole length of the arm and the breast/chest area. Your breast care team will advise you on care of your arm to reduce the risk of lymphoedema – things like looking after your skin and trying to avoid cuts, burns, infections, insect stings and injections on that arm. For more information see Chapter 5.

I've heard that when you have an operation for breast cancer it increases the risk of the cancer spreading. Is this true?

Some people believe this can happen but it has never been proven by research, and breast cancer doctors do not believe it is true. Virtually everyone with breast cancer has surgery and in spite of this breast cancer does not spread in most cases.

If I have a mastectomy, can they rebuild my breast for me?

It is usually possible to rebuild the breast, in what is called a **breast reconstruction**. Sometimes this is done at the same time as the mastectomy, and is called an **immediate reconstruction**; if it's done later it is known as **delayed reconstruction**. This might be a week, months or even years later.

There are several different types of breast reconstruction. You may have an **implant** inserted on its own, or it may be possible to use muscle and tissue from elsewhere in your body. The two usual sites are the top of your back near the shoulder (LD flap) or from your

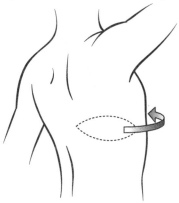

Figure 6 Skin and muscle from the back may be used for breast reconstruction.

abdomen (TRAM or DIEP flap) to replace the mound of the breast, with or without an implant. Two examples are shown in Figures 6 and 7.

More information about the types of breast reconstruction and what they involve can be found in the Breast Cancer Care booklet called *Breast Reconstruction* (see Appendix). Your surgeon and breast care nurse should explain the options you have for reconstruction. You can ask to see photographs of women who have had different types of reconstruction.

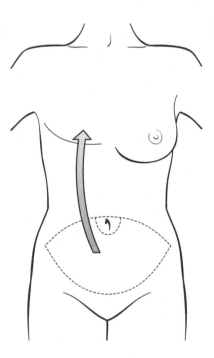

Figure 7 Tissue may be taken from the abdomen
for breast reconstruction.

I am worried about having an implant. Is it safe?

Almost certainly. The DH and many experts in the use of implants have considered the available evidence. They have stated publicly that there is no reason to stop using implants for breast reconstruction surgery. All implants sold within Europe have to pass strict safety checks but will only last an average of 15 years so they may need replacing over time. The Medicines and Healthcare Regulatory Agency (MHRA), the government agency responsible for ensuring that medicines and medical devices are acceptably safe, has published *Information for women considering breast implants* (see Appendix).

Any 'foreign body' implanted into the human body brings the risk of rejection or infection. If you are considering having an implant at the time of your breast surgery, or at a later date, discuss the procedure and its advantages and disadvantages with your surgeon. If you already have an implant and are worried, speak to your surgeon or breast care nurse.

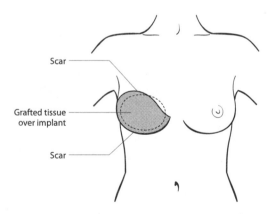

Scar

Grafted tissue
over implant

Scar

Figure 8 Outline of the implant and the possible position of the scar after reconstruction with an implant

If I don't want a breast reconstruction after my mastectomy, can I pad out my bra instead?

Many women choose to use a breast **prosthesis**, which is an artificial breast. It fits in a bra cup or sticks to the chest and replaces all or part of the natural breast shape. While your operation wound heals, you can use a light, soft product temporarily. Then you can have a permanent prosthesis fitted, usually around six weeks later. The NHS hospital where you have your operation will arrange this and give you the prosthesis free of charge. If you have had your surgery in the private sector you may need to pay for your prosthesis, but if you have health insurance, your insurance company may provide it.

There are many different shapes and styles and some different colours to help you find a comfortable fit that closely matches your natural breast. The person fitting you (usually a surgical appliance officer or a breast care nurse) will advise you about caring for and replacing your prosthesis and about best styles of bras and swimming costumes.

If I have a mastectomy, will I look different afterwards?

When you have all your clothes on your appearance and shape shouldn't look different. But when undressed you will see the scars from the mastectomy or the breast reconstruction. If you have a prosthesis, or a reconstructed breast, it will also not move as naturally as the real thing: there will be less 'bounce' when you move and the breast will be more rigid when you lie down. It may also feel less natural to the touch and may not have a nipple. A realistic looking nipple can be created with an operation or by applying an artificial one which sticks onto the breast, but they won't be sensitive to touch or changing temperatures as a natural nipple would.

Everyone is different and for some women decisions about the type of reconstruction or whether to have a nipple, and if so what type, can take some time to make. If you are not sure, don't rush to decide.

Talk to women who have had similar operations or to a counsellor, or your breast care nurse. Make sure that whatever you decide to do is right for you.

If my breasts don't match after surgery, can anything be done?

Yes, you might be able to have an operation on the other side to make the other breast larger or smaller, or to lift it up.

How do I know that what I agree to have done is what will actually happen?

These matters are covered by law. Before your operation your surgeon should explain exactly what he or she proposes to do and why. You will then be asked to sign a consent form which shows that you agree to the operation. In law, the surgeon can only carry out the procedure to which you have consented, unless an emergency arises during the operation and an immediate change of plan is required. This is extremely rare with breast cancer surgery but if such a situation should arise, the surgeon must explain to you what happened and what needed to be done and why.

What will happen before my operation for breast cancer?

This depends on the hospital where you have your operation and the type and extent of breast surgery you are having. You may go into hospital on the day of your operation or the day before. You will meet the doctors, nurses and others who will be caring for you and can ask them any questions you may have about your treatment.

It is normal to be worried before an operation. You are bound to have concerns about what will happen and what the outcome will be. Your breast care nurse can talk with you about it. And there are other people, besides the medical staff, in the hospital who can support you. For example, there are representatives of many religions and faiths who work in or visit hospitals, who are there to listen, and social workers if you are worried about work or finances. Outside the hospital, there are cancer support organisations who give information and support, and you might like to see a counsellor – sometimes just sharing your feelings helps, and talking through fears and concerns with a trained professional can help reduce stress.

What sort of care will I need after my operation?

Again, this depends on the extent of your breast surgery. As you come round from the operation, the nurses will be with you; they will check your pulse and blood pressure fairly often to see how well you are recovering from the anaesthetic.

You would expect there to be some pain or discomfort after an operation, but people experience pain or discomfort in different ways, and again it will depend on the operation you have had. If you feel too sore or uncomfortable you should tell your nurse straight away so you can have some **analgesia** (pain relief). Also tell the nurse if you are feeling sick, so that you can have an **anti-emetic** (anti-sickness) drug.

When you wake up you may have an **intravenous infusion** (an i.v. or 'drip') in your arm which gives you liquid and any drugs you need into a vein. This will only be in place until you start drinking normally again in a day or two.

You may also have tubes to drain the wound of the blood and liquid which result from the surgery. The wound drains remove this liquid from the operation site and help it to heal, and they will be removed after a few days. Sometimes you can go home with the drains still in, and come back to have them taken out at the hospital when you no longer need them.

It could take anything from a few days to a few weeks for your wound to fully heal. Sometimes there is a build-up of liquid near the wound, called a **seroma,** which may drain away naturally or need to be removed by the doctor or nurse with a needle and syringe while you are still in hospital or at a follow-up clinic visit.

Should I keep the arm on the side of the breast surgery still to rest the area?

No, some gentle exercise will actually help the area heal more quickly and get you moving normally again. There are specific exercises you can do, which your surgeon, breast care nurse or a physiotherapist will show you. Find out when to start them and how many times a day you need to do them – it will vary according to the type of operation you have had.

If I have had an operation to cut out the breast cancer, why do I need other treatments as well?

Successful surgery will remove the breast cancer, but cells may have already broken off and travelled elsewhere in the body. Scans and other tests may not be able to detect these very small numbers of cancer cells. Chemotherapy, hormone therapy and targeted therapy reduce the chances of **secondary breast cancer** developing. The cancer can re-grow back in the breast area. Radiotherapy treats the breast area to reduce the risk of this **local recurrence.**

When additional treatments are given as well as surgery, they are called **adjuvant** therapies. Sometimes chemotherapy, hormone therapy or targeted therapy are used before surgery to begin treating the whole body immediately and to shrink the cancer down, making surgery easier. This is called **neo-adjuvant therapy.**

CHEMOTHERAPY

Chemotherapy is the use of drugs to kill abnormal cells. In breast cancer, the aim is to use these drugs to poison cells (called **cytotoxic** drugs) and to destroy any cancer cells that may have spread from the breast to other parts of the body. These cells may not show up in scans or tests, but if you have a type of breast cancer that makes this kind of spread more likely, you could have chemotherapy to make sure your whole body is exposed to these anti-cancer drugs without waiting to see whether or not this will happen in the future.

What's the difference between chemotherapy and radiotherapy?

Chemotherapy is a **systemic** treatment which means it treats all the tissues of the body with anti-cancer drugs. Radiotherapy is a local high-energy X-ray treatment, which only acts in the area of the body where it is given.

Why do some people have radiotherapy and others have chemotherapy?

Actually, many people have both. Like all treatments, the one which will be recommended for you depends on the details of your cancer. Over the years, the progress of people on different treatments is followed up and this research provides cancer specialists with information on when to use chemotherapy and radiotherapy. This way we learn how useful each treatment is, and how to match people to the right treatment, depending on their risk and on which treatments will work best for them.

Chemotherapy may be recommended for people whose breast cancer is large, high grade or has spread to the lymph glands, for example. Radiotherapy may be more suitable for those who have had breast conservation surgery to treat the remaining breast tissue and reduce the chances of the breast cancer coming back there or in some cases to the chest wall after mastectomy, depending on whether the lymph nodes contain cancer cells.

Will I have chemotherapy after my surgery?

It depends on your individual course of treatment, based on the features of your cancer. It is most common to have chemotherapy after surgery as an adjuvant, or additional treatment, and if this is the plan, it might start about three to six weeks after surgery to allow you to get over the operation. Some people have neo-adjuvant treatment to shrink a large tumour before the operation. If you have secondary breast cancer, chemotherapy may be the only treatment to be suggested. You can discuss all this with your doctor or breast care nurse.

I don't understand how chemotherapy can stop the cancer from growing. What do these drugs do?

Chemotherapy drugs aim to destroy cancer cells by interfering with their ability to grow and divide. Each drug does this in a different way so most people have a combination of two or three (either one at a time or all together) to attack the cancer cells in several ways to increase the chances of killing them.

I am about to start my course of chemotherapy. What will actually happen?

The most common way is an injection into a vein using a syringe or through a 'drip'. This means being in the hospital for about half a day as you need to have blood tests and wait for the results of these before each treatment.

Will I have the same drugs as other people having chemotherapy for breast cancer?

Not necessarily. There are at least six different combinations used to treat people with primary breast cancer: that is a cancer that is only in the breast but may have spread to the lymph nodes. There are also other drugs which are used for secondary breast cancer, which has spread to other parts of the body. Drugs are usually used in combination to increase the chances of killing the most cancer cells (see question above).

These single drugs and combinations are often used in primary breast cancer:

- FEC (5fluorouracil, epirubicin and cyclophosphamide);
- CMF (cyclophosphamide, methotrexate and 5fluorouracil);
- epirubicin then CMF;
- FEC then docetaxel (Taxotere®);
- AC: Adriamycin® (doxorubicin), cyclophosphamide.
- TAC: Taxotere® (docetaxel), Adriamycin® (doxorubicin), cyclophosphamide.

These drugs are usually used to treat secondary breast cancer:

- capecitabine (Xeloda®);
- vinorelbine (Navelbine®);
- gemcitabine (Gemzar®).

I need to plan ahead to organise my work, the children and so on. How long does a course of chemotherapy for breast cancer usually take?

It depends on the exact combination you are having but it is usually several months. Normally, you would be given between four and eight doses in total every three or four weeks. Between each treatment your body can rest and recover before the next one – a 'rest period'. You don't usually need to visit hospital between treatments (unless you need help with side effects) but you will need a blood test before each treatment to see how your body is coping.

Won't the cancer cells continue growing between treatments?

It's unlikely, as the effect of the drugs carries on for quite a few days after the treatment has been given. Cancer cells don't recover as quickly as normal cells, so repeating the treatments gradually reduces the total number of cancer cells that are, or may be, present in your body.

My doctor says my chemotherapy is an 'insurance policy'. What does this mean?

It means that chemotherapy is reducing the risk of your cancer spreading. Because tests and scans often can't detect breast cancer cells that have spread through the body, adjuvant (additional) chemotherapy is given as a precaution in case they have spread. Chemotherapy can reduce the risk of cancer from coming back, and your doctor will know how long chemotherapy needs to be given in order to be most effective.

If my breast cancer comes back, will I be able to have more chemotherapy treatment?

Yes, but you may be given a different combination of drugs, depending on which ones you had before and how long you had them for.

You hear stories about how awful chemotherapy is. Are there lots of side effects?

Not always. Some people experience few side effects during chemotherapy and are able to carry on with daily life more or less as usual. For others, chemotherapy is a miserable experience which has a considerable effect on their lives.

It isn't always helpful to listen to other people's experiences of chemotherapy as effects can vary so much. It depends not only on which of the many drugs you have, but also on your own individual reaction to the drugs: two people receiving the same combination of drugs may feel completely different during their courses of treatment.

Why do chemotherapy drugs usually cause side effects?

Chemotherapy drugs destroy cells which are constantly and rapidly dividing – which is the way cancer cells behave. But normal, healthy cells grow and divide rapidly to repair body tissues, and so these cells will be damaged too. It is this damage which causes side effects. As chemotherapy is a **systemic** treatment, this means that side effects are also systemic and so affect body systems such as the digestive system and the **immune system**. Fortunately, normal cells recover quickly so any side effects of treatment are usually temporary. Most people have at least some side effects, but it will depend on the drugs you are having. The doctors and nurses will advise you on what to expect, and also on how to cope with any side effects. Some of the more common side effects are dealt with in the following questions.

I've been told that once I start treatment I will have to have regular blood tests. Why is this necessary?

The blood tests are to check the amount of red and white blood cells in your blood. Chemotherapy can slow down production of healthy amounts of both red and white blood cells. If this happens, you are more at risk of infections (because of too few **white blood cells**) and **anaemia** (too few **red blood cells**). Regular blood tests will show if the drugs are affecting your **blood count**. You might need some treatment, such as antibiotics for an infection or a blood transfusion for anaemia. If the blood count is low, the doctors can either adjust the dose of your drugs or lengthen your rest period between treatments. Although it is worrying and frustrating when this happens, it isn't unusual. It is much safer to delay treatment by about a week than to give the drugs before your body has recovered.

When they take a blood sample, what are they actually looking for?

Three types of blood cells are each measured:

- **white blood cells** which help fight infection;
- **platelets** which help the blood to clot, preventing bleeding and bruising; and
- **red blood cells** which carry oxygen to all the body's tissues.

What does it mean if I have a low blood count or if my blood count falls?

Very often you won't notice anything unusual. Sometimes people say that they feel a bit depressed and tired when their count is at its lowest about 10–14 days after treatment. However, if your count has dropped, or is expected to, you may be told to look out for certain signs or symptoms which should be reported to your doctor.

What kind of things might indicate that my blood count is low?

When your white cells are low, you will be more likely to develop an infection. You should contact your doctor if you have a sore throat or start running a high temperature, or if you notice anything else that might mean you have an infection, such as a burning sensation when you pass urine.

A drop in your platelet count will mean you may bruise more easily. You might notice that your gums bleed when you brush your teeth, or you might have a nosebleed.

If your red blood cells are affected, you may become anaemic and may feel tired or short of breath, although this is rare.

It is very important that you report anything unusual for you to the doctor or your breast care nurse straight away, even if it seems trivial, so that the doctors can check you out and treat you if necessary before it becomes more serious. Everyone having chemotherapy is given a list of emergency contact numbers so you can get in touch with someone from your team if you need to.

Is there anything that can stop my blood count falling too low while I have chemotherapy?

You may have an injection of G-CSF if you are having certain combinations of chemotherapy drugs, or if your blood count is low at each treatment. G-CSF stands for **granulocyte-colony stimulating factors**, and it helps increase the number of white cells being produced during chemotherapy. This means that you can have your chemotherapy as usual without lengthened rest periods in between.

If I need a blood transfusion, is there a risk of catching AIDS?

Virtually none. All donor blood is tested for the HIV virus, which causes AIDS, and people in known high-risk groups are discouraged from giving blood. In addition, blood products are heat treated to destroy the virus. The risk of transfer of the disease in this way is very small indeed.

Will I feel sick when I am on chemotherapy?

You may feel sick, or occasionally even vomit, after some types of chemotherapy drugs. This can last for one to five days after each treatment, but it may be longer. There are many anti-emetic (anti-sickness) drugs you can take during your treatment, or straight afterwards, to reduce any nausea or vomiting. It is best to take these regularly as prescribed rather than wait until you feel sick.

The staff caring for you may also have other suggestions to reduce sickness, such as changes in eating patterns and learning relaxation techniques.

Part of my chemotherapy is in the form of tablets. Will these make me feel sick?

Possibly – you may find taking the tablets at night will solve this problem. Check with your doctor if you can do this.

If one anti-sickness drug doesn't work, can I try another?

Yes. Tell the doctor or nurse before your next treatment. There are several drugs which can be prescribed.

Will the chemotherapy I'm having make my hair fall out?

It depends on what chemotherapy drugs you are having but most of them cause at least some hair loss. The hair may get thinner or fall out in patches. You may also lose your eyelashes and eyebrows. Treat your hair gently to help keep it in good condition: don't have it coloured or permed and use a cool setting on the hairdryer or heated rollers. Try to avoid anything that can damage your hair, such as brushing it hard or plaiting it. Always ask for advice if you are in any doubt about what to do.

Is there anything I can try to stop the hair loss?

Some people choose to try something called scalp cooling. This involves wearing a very cold hat before, during and after each treatment to try and reduce blood flow to the scalp, so the drugs don't reach the hair roots and damage them. It doesn't work for everyone and can be uncomfortable, but you can ask your doctor or breast care nurse about trying it.

Will my hair grow back after my chemotherapy?

Hair loss from chemotherapy is always temporary and the hair grows back in the months after treatment. You may even find your hair starts to re-grow before the end of the course of chemotherapy.

When my hair grows back will it be the same as before?

Not necessarily: sometimes the hair grows back a different colour or texture than before. It may be curly instead of straight. It is not possible to predict whether this will happen to you.

If I'm going to lose my hair, how soon will it happen and what can I do about it?

It could be a few days or a few weeks before your hair begins to fall out. You will probably notice more hair in your brush or comb. There may be hair on your pillow in the morning, which may upset you – wearing a hairnet or turban overnight may help how you feel about this. Some people prefer to cut their hair short or shave their heads as soon as the hair starts coming out. Your hospital can arrange for you to be fitted with a wig before your treatment starts, but if you don't want to wear a wig, a cap, hat or scarf is an alternative.

You will need to wear something on your head to protect your scalp from the cold, and in the sun you must have a hat and sunblock cream. If your scalp becomes dry, use a gentle moisturiser.

Will the chemotherapy make me lose my body hair?

Some drugs do cause temporary loss of all body hair. Ask if this is expected in your case.

Is having chemotherapy painful and does it always have to be given through a 'drip' in the hand or arm?

Chemotherapy may be no more painful than having an injection or a blood test. However, as the course of treatment goes on the drugs can make your veins at, and above, the injection site more

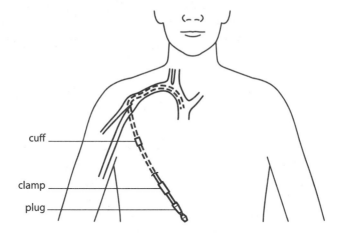

Figure 9 A Hickman line

sensitive or sore. You should tell your doctor or nurse if this happens so the sore areas can be avoided.

Sometimes the veins are severely affected by the drugs and become hard to find so that injections become very difficult. If this happens you may be offered an **intravenous (IV) catheter** (tube) which stays in place until the chemotherapy has finished. For example, a **central venous catheter** (a 'Hickman line') is passed underneath the skin of the chest into a large vein just above the heart. Another type, called a **peripherally inserted central catheter** (PICC), is inserted into one of the large veins in the arm until it also sits in a large vein above the heart. A third alternative is an **implanted port** (Portcath®) when a catheter is passed under the skin of the chest into a large vein above the heart, but a port remains under the skin and a special needle is used to inject into this when needed.

These kinds of catheter can be left in place for many months. Drugs and fluids can be given through them and blood samples can also be taken from them. To stop them blocking, they need regular weekly flushing with **saline** (sterile salt water) using a syringe. This can be done by either a district nurse or a friend or partner after training. The dressing covering where they enter the body will need changing regularly to prevent any infection. An implanted port does not need a dressing once the wound has healed.

Why do some people have a Hickman line or PICC and others don't?

Many people simply don't need one because their veins remain fine during a course of breast cancer chemotherapy.

Can I eat and drink normally during chemotherapy?

Yes. You may find you lose your appetite for a few days after your treatment but when it returns to normal you can eat your usual foods. Try to drink more while you are having chemotherapy to make sure you are well-hydrated, especially if you are being sick. Generally, it is fine to have alcoholic drinks but some chemotherapy drugs can affect your taste, and for a while you may no longer enjoy certain foods or drinks. If you have any problems with eating tell your doctor or nurse. They may be able to offer some suggestions or ask the hospital dietitian to advise you.

Can chemotherapy affect my chances of having children?

In women, chemotherapy can affect the healthy development of eggs, which in turn can affect fertility. If you have not yet started or completed your family, this can be a major issue, and you will need to think about it carefully. Sometimes periods become irregular or stop during chemotherapy, but this may be temporary and doesn't mean you cannot conceive. However, in some women periods don't come back and it is no longer possible to become pregnant. This is more likely the older you are when you start treatment, because you are nearer to the natural age of menopause.

Talk to your doctors and breast care nurses about what you might expect from treatment and tell them if you plan to have children. They can discuss any options with you and may refer you to a specialist fertility doctor to explore these options in more depth before your treatment begins.

It is essential not to become pregnant during or immediately after chemotherapy as the fetus could be affected, so you must use an effective form of contraception throughout treatment, though not the Pill because it contains hormones that could affect your breast cancer.

Can I father a child after I've had chemotherapy?

Men with breast cancer can also have problems with fertility, though it is not common. If you plan to father a child in the future discuss this with your doctor before you start your treatment. If your treatment is likely to make you permanently sterile, you should be offered an opportunity to 'bank' sperm before starting treatment. Once again, use contraception during and after chemotherapy.

My daughter is getting married soon and the date coincides with my chemotherapy. Can I change the day of my injection?

Usually the doctors are quite willing to change treatment dates by a few days to fit in with special occasions like a wedding, or so you can have a short holiday, so do ask if you can reorganise your dates.

Will I see the doctor regularly during treatment?

Every time you come to hospital for chemotherapy you will usually see a doctor or a nurse who will want to know how you feel and how the chemotherapy is affecting you. Talk about anything unusual you may have experienced, whether it was expected or not. Use this time to discuss any worries you may have and to ask questions. Don't worry if it's a physical change or a concern that seems trivial – it's always best to check. Ask the doctor before taking other medicines and, if you wish to try a **complementary therapy**, find out if there is any reason why you should not use it at this time.

RADIOTHERAPY

Radiotherapy is the use of high-energy X-rays, in this case to destroy any cancer cells that may have been left behind in the breast area after surgery.

Radiotherapy also reaches normal cells which are in the treatment area. All cells are more vulnerable to damage when they are dividing. Cancer cells divide more rapidly than normal cells so will be damaged or killed at a greater rate than the normal cells in the treatment area. Any normal cells that are affected by radiotherapy recover or repair themselves more easily.

But radiation can cause cancer: how can it be used to treat it?

Radiation may cause cancer if someone is exposed to large doses in a very short time period. When radiation is used as radiotherapy it is very carefully controlled. The beam of rays is directed exactly, and only, at the area needing treatment. The dose of radiation is relatively small and is given over a period of weeks. When radiation causes cancer it is due to someone being exposed to a very high dose in a short period of time, such as the very rare instances when someone is close to a leak in a nuclear power plant.

Can I have radiotherapy instead of an operation?

No, radiotherapy would not be effective enough to treat the breast cancer if used on its own. It is usually recommended after any type of breast conserving surgery and after mastectomy if cancer cells are seen in the lymph nodes under your arm, to reduce the chances of the breast cancer coming back. If you are not having chemotherapy, you will ideally start radiotherapy within a few weeks of surgery. If you are having chemotherapy, then the radiotherapy will usually follow this.

Is radiotherapy painful?

Having the treatment is painless but it can have a few side effects that are described in answers later in this section. Most side effects of radiotherapy for breast cancer occur towards the end of the course of treatment and may continue for a few weeks afterwards.

How is radiotherapy given?

Radiotherapy is given using machines that produce X-rays that are beamed directly at the breast/chest area (see Figure 10).

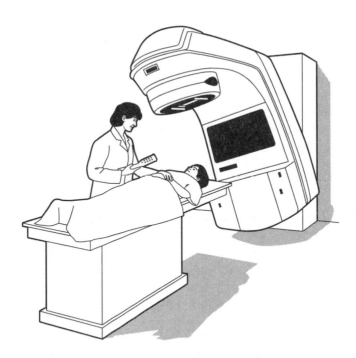

Figure 10 Having radiotherapy

How long does radiotherapy last? Will I just have one treatment?

Radiotherapy to the breast or chest area is usually given as a course of treatment lasting three to six weeks. There are usually between three and five treatments each week, normally on weekdays. The actual treatment only lasts for a few minutes, but before each one you, and the machine, have to be carefully placed in the right position by the radiographers, and this often takes longer than the treatment itself.

If you are having radiotherapy to treat secondary breast cancer in the bones or brain, the course of treatment will be shorter, lasting only a few days.

I've been told I have to attend for 'planning' before starting my treatment. What is this?

Planning is an essential part of your radiotherapy, and will make sure the treatment is accurate. Your treatment planning involves working out the exact dose of radiotherapy you need and precisely where in your body it needs to go. The radiotherapy beam must be directed accurately to hit the right area but to avoid unnecessarily hitting healthy tissue with X-rays. In the planning session a **simulator** will create a mock-up of treatment using measurements or scans or both. The planning phase may take an hour or more.

After all this preparation, how can the doctors be sure that treatment is identical each day I have it?

When the doctors have decided on the exact area to be treated, it will be marked out on your skin. These marks can then be used to line up the machine each time so that the correct area is treated. They will use either an indelible pen or a permanent pinprick tattoo. Although indelible, the pen will not be permanent so don't wash it off during the course of treatment. The tattoo is permanent but should be small enough as to be almost invisible to anyone not looking for it.

Am I radioactive during a course of radiotherapy?

Certainly not. The machine emitting X-rays is only on for the treatment time and is switched off afterwards. There is no radiation left in you or in the air around you when the machine has been switched off at the end of your treatment.

Do I need to stay overnight in hospital for radiotherapy?

No, radiotherapy is given as an outpatient treatment.

What will actually happen when I go for my radiotherapy treatment?

Every day's treatment routine is the same. When you enter the radiotherapy room you'll be asked to undress to the waist so that the marked out area is visible. You'll lie down like you did in the simulator and the radiographers, who supervise and deliver your treatment, will use light beams to help position you correctly. When you are in the correct position, they will ask you to remain very still, although you can breathe and swallow normally. They will leave the room and switch on the radiotherapy machine. For a very short time you will be on your own, but the radiographers will be able to see you all the time on a closed-circuit television, and you can talk to each other via a microphone system.

The radiographers work with radiotherapy daily and it is important that they are not exposed to unnecessary radiation. This is why they cannot stay with you.

As your treatment goes on you will get used to this procedure. If you have any questions or concerns, talk to the radiographers who will advise you. They understand that at first this is a frightening experience for most people.

Will the radiotherapy give me radiation sickness?

No. 'Radiation sickness' describes a whole series of symptoms which people experience when they have been exposed to large amounts of radiation after major nuclear accidents, such as the Chernobyl disaster. Radiotherapy to the breast or chest area doesn't cause nausea or vomiting or any of the symptoms associated with radiation sickness.

Will radiotherapy make my hair fall out?

Radiotherapy causes hair loss only in the area being treated. So a woman having radiotherapy to the breast won't lose any hair on her head. Men being treated for breast cancer can lose chest hair. You will lose your underarm hair with radiotherapy to the armpit. Hair loss from radiotherapy can be permanent.

Radiotherapy causes sore skin, doesn't it?

The radiotherapy burns that people once talked about are very rarely seen now. Research is going on to find the best way of giving radiotherapy with the fewest side effects. Sometimes your skin may become sore and you may get symptoms such as redness, skin darkening, itching or moist, weepy skin. Always follow the radiographers' advice about the care of your skin.

Apart from sore skin, what other kind of side effects am I likely to experience during radiotherapy?

Some people feel extremely tired towards the end of their treatment, and for a few weeks or even months afterwards. But often you can carry on your usual life and even go to work if you choose.

If part of your **oesophagus** (gullet) is in the treatment area, you may have difficulty swallowing towards the end of treatment. This is because the cells in that area can be affected by repeated doses of X-rays and gradually lose their ability to recover between the daily doses. Any discomfort usually goes away within a week or two of the end of the course of treatment.

Will I have any long-term side effects after my course of radiotherapy?

In the longer term the skin over the breast may remain reddened and the breast may be slightly swollen. Also, the area under the skin that has been treated can feel hard and sometimes be uncomfortable. This is because of **fibrosis** which is similar to scar tissue, and can happen some months – or even years – after treatment. In severe cases it can distort the shape of the breast and may also lead to lymphoedema (swelling) by blocking the lymph drainage of the arm (see p. 113).

Rarely, the radiotherapy can damage parts of the body near to the area being treated. In breast cancer treatment, this would be the lung, the heart (if it is the left breast) and the ribs. For most people any such damage will gradually heal.

Will I see a doctor during my course of radiotherapy?

Yes, you will probably see a radiotherapy doctor (called a **radiotherapist** or **clinical oncologist**) each week or two. If you are worried about anything during treatment, take the opportunity to discuss it with your doctor, radiographer or breast care nurse.

Is there anything that I shouldn't do during radiotherapy treatment?

You will be told if there is anything specific you should or shouldn't do, but here is a list of general points.

- **Do** look after yourself, eat well and have plenty to drink, especially water.

- **Do** make sure you get lots of rest. You might be able to carry on as usual but, on the other hand, you may find you can only work part-time or you may need help with shopping or housework.

- **Do** wear comfortable clothes. If you have treatment marks on your skin you might prefer to wear older clothes so new things are not marked by the ink. Loose-fitting underwear and clothes are best, as they won't rub on the treatment area and make your skin sore.

- **Do** take notice of the skin care advice the radiographers give you, especially about whether or not you can use any creams or lotions. The ink marks must not be washed off but you will usually be able to splash tepid water on your skin and gently pat it dry to keep yourself feeling clean.

- **Do** follow your breast care nurse's advice about wearing a breast prosthesis during treatment. You will usually be advised to wear a 'comfy' or post-operative one in order to avoid any skin irritation.

- **Do** keep your treatment area out of the sun and cold winds, and don't use hot-water bottles or ice packs. Your skin will be more sensitive than usual.

- **Do** ask if you are unsure about anything, or have specific concerns about your personal treatment or side effects.

HORMONE (ENDOCRINE) THERAPY

Hormones are like messengers: along with the system of nerves, they regulate everything our bodies automatically do. Hormones are made in **endocrine glands** (such as the thyroid and adrenal glands) and they work by attaching to receptors on target cells. There are many hormones, including oestrogen and progesterone which control a woman's menstrual cycle, for example.

Hormone therapy is a drug treatment which aims to prevent the hormone oestrogen from stimulating the breast cancer to grow. This kind of treatment is sometimes called **endocrine therapy**.

My doctor has recommended I have hormone therapy. How does this work?

Some breast cancers are stimulated to grow by the hormone oestrogen. Hormone therapies block oestrogen, preventing it from having any effect on breast cancer cells. They do this by stopping the hormone from attaching to the breast cancer cells or by lowering the overall amount of oestrogen in the body.

My friend didn't have hormone therapy for her breast cancer, though I am. Why do some people have this treatment and not others?

Hormone therapy will only suit you if your breast cancer has receptors on its cell surface that latch on to hormones and use them to help it grow faster. This kind of cancer is called **oestrogen** or **progesterone receptor positive breast cancer**. Progesterone is another hormone whose receptors indicate that oestrogen is being used to help the cancer grow. Like chemotherapy, hormone therapy is a systemic treatment because it can reach cancer cells anywhere in the body. The usual time to have hormone therapy is as an additional treatment after surgery and chemotherapy, or during or just after radiotherapy. It is quite common to have both chemotherapy and hormone therapy because the features of the cancer indicate that both will offer benefits.

Will having hormone therapy mean I need to have regular injections?

Most hormone therapies involve taking tablets once a day. There are one or two which are given by an injection into the tummy muscles, usually once a month.

How long will I be taking hormone therapy?

If you have primary breast cancer, the hormone therapy usually lasts for five years. People taking hormone therapy for secondary breast cancer usually stay on it indefinitely, unless it is no longer effective at controlling the cancer.

My friend is on a different hormone therapy to me. Why would this be?

There are several hormone therapies used to treat breast cancer. They include:

- tamoxifen;
- anastrozole (Arimidex®);
- letrozole (Femara®);
- exemestane (Aromasin®);
- goserelin (Zoladex®);
- fulvestrant (Faslodex®).

Some hormone therapies only work after or before the menopause, so the drug you have will depend on this, and also whether you have primary or secondary breast cancer. The doctor will also have to bear in mind any hormone therapies you may have had before.

Am I likely to get any side effects from hormone therapy?

Yes, and they will depend on which hormone you are taking. If your doctor recommends hormone therapy, ask what specific side effects you should expect. Generally side effects are similar to menopausal symptoms, such as hot flushes, night sweats, dry skin and mood swings. Some people also experience weight gain and some of the drugs cause joint pain. These often get better after taking the drug for some months. Do tell your doctor or breast care nurse about any side effects because they may be able to suggest ways of relieving them.

I was taking hormone replacement therapy. Is this the same as hormone therapy?

No, hormone replacement therapy (HRT) is used to treat symptoms women have at the time of the menopause. It is completely different as it supplies hormones to the body rather than preventing them from forming or working. It is not used in the treatment of breast cancer.

TARGETED THERAPY

This is a more recent type of therapy which has only been used widely over the last few years. The drugs work by blocking the different ways that breast cancer cells grow and develop. They are different to chemotherapy and hormone therapies.

Herceptin® (trastuzumab) is the most well-known **targeted therapy**. It works by blocking a protein (HER-2) that stimulates breast cancer cells to grow. Herceptin is given as an infusion in a drip into a vein in the hand or arm. You may have it on its own, at the time you are having chemotherapy (and continuing afterwards) or after chemotherapy has finished.

I have just started on Herceptin. How long will I be on it?

Each dose takes between 30 and 90 minutes to give, and you receive it in an outpatient department or day care unit every three weeks. The best length of time to be on Herceptin is not yet certain, but if you have primary breast cancer you will usually be on it for about a year.

Should I expect any side effects while I'm having Herceptin?

Herceptin is different to chemotherapy and does not cause sickness or hair loss. Common side effects include flu-like symptoms, such as fever and chills, nausea and diarrhoea. These are usually worst on the first or second infusions but improve over time. In very rare cases, Herceptin can affect the way your heart works, so the heart is monitored with regular scans throughout the treatment. This means that if you have any problems they can be spotted early on, and the treatment can be stopped if necessary to allow the heart to recover.

> *I'm not sure about Herceptin. Are there any other targeted cancer therapies?*

New targeted therapies are being studied in **clinical trials** but at the time of writing they have not been licensed or approved for routine use within the UK. More will probably be available to treat primary and secondary breast cancer within the coming months and years.

> *If the treatment for my breast cancer doesn't work or my cancer comes back after my treatment, what happens then?*

It will depend when and where the breast cancer comes back, but you will almost certainly be advised to have more treatment. This may be further surgery, another course of radiotherapy, more chemotherapy or a different type of hormone therapy. You may be asked to try new treatments that are being assessed as part of a clinical trial.

CLINICAL TRIALS

A clinical trial is a research study, in which two or more groups of patients are given different treatments and the results compared. Trials are used to investigate:

- new treatments for cancer;
- different ways of giving care;
- treatments used to relieve symptoms.

A trial may compare a new treatment with the best standard treatment currently available. Two methods of giving the same treatment may be tested against each other. Much of what is now accepted as standard treatment was tested in this way. Doctors rely on the results of clinical trials when they suggest or advise you about treatment.

Clinical trials have helped us make many advances in the diagnosis and treatment of breast cancer. Most of the newer drugs have been developed and introduced into everyday treatment as a result of such trials. Until recently the general term 'research' was used, so many people think these trials are new. (Clinical trials are one specific type of research.)

How will I know if I'm in a clinical trial?

By law, your doctor must tell you at the very beginning that the treatment option being recommended for you is being evaluated as part of a clinical trial or a research study. One of the questions you might like to ask your doctor is 'Is this a trial?' or 'Is this a research project?' If any of the other staff caring for you, such as the nurses, are conducting a study of any kind you should also be informed.

Do I have to give my permission before I can be entered into a trial?

Yes. The staff running the trial must have your consent before they can do anything to you. You sign a consent form before an operation and many hospitals now ask for your written consent before some investigations, and before a course of radiotherapy or chemotherapy. You must agree to what the doctors, or other staff, propose before they can proceed. This is even more important if you

are being asked to enter a clinical trial.

I'm thinking about taking part in a new drug trial. What should I know about the research?

There are several things you should be told, for example:

- what the trial involves;
- what benefits you may expect from it;
- what side effects might occur; and
- what it means to you in the way of extra tests or visits to hospital, and so on.

You will be given some written information and allowed time to decide whether or not to join the trial. There may be more questions you want to ask in order to understand what is planned. You should not give your consent until you are completely happy about the project.

There is a new drug trial which my doctor sounds keen on. I have read all the papers about it, but I'm not sure. What if I say no?

You have the right to say yes or no to any treatment which is suggested. If you do not wish to take part in a trial you should say so. It will not affect your current or future treatment or care in any way. Your doctor will then discuss with you any other treatments that are available.

If I do decide to join the drug trial, what happens if I change my mind later?

You can withdraw from the trial at any time without having to give a reason. You can then discuss different treatment options with your doctor. On the other hand, if you originally decided not to take part, and later change your mind, you can discuss this with your doctor.

Are there different types of trials?

Yes. There are many different ways in which trials are organised and several methods of analysing statistics or information. Organisations like **Breast Cancer Care** and **Cancerbackup**, among others, produce information about clinical trials (see Appendix for contact details).

How do I find out if there is a trial being run somewhere else which might benefit me?

First of all, ask your doctor who may know of research being carried out in a regional cancer centre or specialist hospital. Second, if you have heard about a trial in another hospital you can contact them directly. You will usually need a referral letter from your cancer specialist or GP in order to be seen by the doctors doing the trial. And finally, you might be able to find out from one of the cancer information services, such as Cancer Research UK (addresses in Appendix).

In terms of a clinical trial, what does 'eligible' mean?

It means that you fall into a strictly-defined group of people needed for this particular trial. When the doctors design a clinical trial, they have to lay down clear guidelines about who is included. For example, a trial of a drug for post-menopausal women won't give useful results if some of the women are much younger. If you don't come within the guidelines you will not be able to take part in the trial. So you may not be eligible for a trial even if it's of a new treatment for the same kind of breast cancer that you have.

Can't I get the new treatment if I'm able to pay for it?

No, offering to pay will make no difference if a clinical trial is being used to test or evaluate a new treatment.

MAKING CHOICES

If I go as a private patient from the start of my treatment, will I get better care and a better range of treatment choices?

Generally you will get equally good treatment and care within the NHS. In some regional cancer centres you may find a wider range of NHS services than are available privately. Private care may offer such benefits as always seeing your consultant at appointments, and getting to know a smaller team of staff. The majority of staff on teams offering private care also work within the NHS. It is a good idea to check that a private hospital has been approved as a breast unit.

If I am undecided about treatment or not satisfied with my treatment can I get a second opinion?

Yes. Many breast unit teams will positively encourage you in seeking a second opinion. Discuss this with your hospital doctor. You will need a letter of referral to another specialist from either your current specialist or GP.

If your hospital doctor is unhappy about your request, see your family doctor who can also refer you on for another opinion. Most doctors are sympathetic in this situation. They understand that when faced with a diagnosis of cancer everyone wants to have the best treatment for themselves or their family.

4 | Complementary therapies

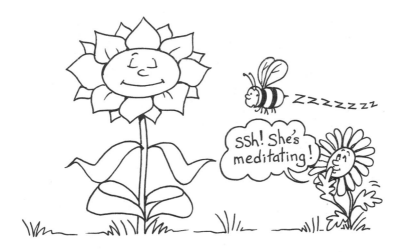

This chapter answers some of the most common questions people with breast cancer ask about the use of complementary therapies, and explains some of the therapies in a little more detail. Please remember that there is no reliable scientific evidence to show that any of the therapies listed can either cure breast cancer or control it. Having said that, many people find that using them helps them to improve their 'quality of life', that is their physical, emotional, spiritual and psychological well-being. There has been limited research into the effectiveness of most complementary therapies. Conventional medicine relies on clinical trials to find out if a treatment works and the 'gold standard' of these is a randomised trial, where one treatment is compared to another – or no treatment at all (see Chapter 3). Because of the lack of this type of research it is impossible to say whether a specific therapy may benefit people with breast cancer.

You can get more information about the therapies mentioned in this chapter by contacting the relevant national association or organisation – addresses are listed in the Appendix.

Many support groups or support centres offer complementary therapies. Sometimes therapies are free or you may be asked for a donation according to what you can afford. Other centres charge a fee. If you see a private therapist, check their fees beforehand as well as their qualifications.

What are complementary therapies?

Complementary therapies are, as the name suggests, treatments or therapies that may complement or supplement the 'conventional' medical treatments already described in Chapter 3. You might find one or more of these therapies useful in reducing the amount of stress you feel, or in helping you to relax during or after your treatment. They are also sometimes referred to as 'supportive' therapies.

Many complementary therapies require you to take an active part, so you feel you are doing something to help yourself. For some people, using one or more complementary therapies gives them a sense of taking control, as it is a part of their treatment which they have chosen to use rather than had prescribed for them.

What's the difference between complementary therapies and alternative therapies?

Complementary therapies used to be called alternative therapies. This implied that they should be used instead of 'conventional' medical treatments. The change in name reflects a change in attitude: they are now seen as additional, rather than separate, options. Some people do still refer to alternative therapies when they mean using therapies instead of using conventional medicine. In this book we are *not* advocating this approach.

Sometimes alternative therapies are called 'unproven' therapies.

This means that no formal research has been published to show their effectiveness, and this is why health professionals often suggest people avoid them during their cancer treatment.

Can I use alternative or complementary therapies instead of having hospital treatment?

Yes, if you wish to but you should discuss the pros and cons fully with your surgeon, oncologist and breast care nurse. This is an important decision and, as stated at the beginning of this chapter, there is no reliable evidence that any alternative or complementary therapy can cure or control breast cancer.

Are there many complementary therapies to choose from?

Dozens! But those that may be particularly helpful for people who have breast cancer are described in this chapter.

Do complementary therapies work?

That's a question that doesn't have a direct answer. Some people swear by one method. Others try one or more therapies during and after they have had surgery, radiotherapy or chemotherapy. Not everyone will find that they benefit from using complementary therapies, but for many people the option to at least try is all-important.

It is perhaps worth mentioning that not everyone wants to use complementary therapies. No one should be pushed into trying something they are not sure about just because a relative or friend is convinced it would be helpful.

How could these therapies help me?

Many complementary therapies take an **holistic** approach. This means that you are seen as a whole person in terms of your physical body, your mind and your spirit. Many conventional doctors and nurses also try to take a holistic approach. Physical symptoms you might be experiencing from your cancer or your treatment are taken into account together with your feelings and emotions. So it's not simply a question having treatment given to a particular part of you. Rather, it involves letting a practitioner know how you are feeling in a broader sense, in order that you can work together to face the cancer and any treatment and side effects you might experience. The therapies are unlikely to completely remove the side effects of some treatments, but you might find they reduce those you do have.

Therapies which focus on your emotional and psychological well-being may be aimed at stimulating your immune system by helping you to relax and so reduce any stress or tension you might have. These therapies give you a central role in your own treatment and can encourage a positive outlook. Feeling you are doing something to help yourself can give you a tremendous boost.

Will my doctor refuse to treat me if I use complementary therapies?

No doctor should refuse to treat a person who wishes to use complementary therapies alongside hospital treatment, as long as the therapies used are not likely to interfere with the hospital treatment or to make any side effects worse. The majority of cancer specialists now accept that many of their patients use therapies that aim to provide emotional and psychological support. They may, however, be less keen on other therapies. If you find this to be so you should ask why, in case there are valid medical reasons against your choice.

If I decide to use a particular complementary therapy, do I still have to go back to the doctor for regular check-ups?

Yes, regular check-ups are important, as without them your progress cannot be properly monitored. So you should continue going to see whoever is in charge of your aftercare – either the doctor at the hospital follow-up clinic or your family doctor.

How do I choose a therapy that's right for me?

Choosing between therapies can be very difficult. You could:

- talk to others who have used them;
- contact some of the organisations listed in the Appendix for information;
- visit centres where different therapies are practised;
- read books about them.

Then try one or more that you find appealing.

Does the kind of breast cancer I have make a difference to the therapy I choose?

It should be considered, as some therapies might not be helpful in certain cases. For example, some herbal remedies might not be prescribed if your breast cancer is hormone receptor positive (see Chapter 3). You should tell the therapist what type of breast cancer you have and what other treatment you are having or have had, even if it is some time ago.

A fully qualified and experienced therapist will take an extensive history of your breast cancer, and any other medical conditions, before developing a therapy plan for you. It may be that the therapy you are interested in is not suitable for you because of a possible interaction with your treatment. It is also very important you tell your therapist what medicines you are taking.

If you are still having treatment or regular check-ups at a hospital, you might also want to ask the opinion of one of the health professionals there.

Does my hospital treatment affect my choice of complementary therapy?

Yes, it does (see previous question). Some hospital treatments cause side effects that might be made worse if a particular therapy is being used at the same time. For example, if you are having chemotherapy treatment that causes you to be feel sick or to vomit, the hospital staff might suggest a type of diet you should eat to try to reduce this side effect. It's not a good idea to introduce a completely new complementary diet at this time. If you are having radiotherapy, massage to the area being treated is not a good idea during the weeks of treatment, and for a few weeks afterwards, because of the sensitivity of your skin. However, you could have massage to another part of your body.

How do I know if a therapist would be suitable to work with me?

A qualified therapist shouldn't take you on as a client without first knowing all the relevant facts about you. If you are not asked directly you should tell the therapist about your breast cancer and any treatment you have had. If s/he then feels that the therapy might be unsuitable for you, it is unlikely that they will suggest you start to work with them. A good therapist should advise you against a therapy that might adversely affect your breast cancer or 'conventional' treatment.

Do all therapists have recognised qualifications?

Many types of complementary therapy require therapists to belong to national or professional associations, specific for different therapies. Each association should be concerned with training, qualifications, and/or accreditation schemes, and they should not permit any member to practise if they have not satisfied some specific criteria or are not suitably qualified. In addition, the professional associations supporting most of the therapies listed in this chapter require their members to undertake continuing professional development courses to update their knowledge and skills in order to remain registered. So it is essential to check that the person you are planning to see has reached a recognised standard, for example a diploma or degree in their therapy. Simply having a certificate on the wall is not always a guarantee of expertise.

For example, a person can claim to be a counsellor even if they have only completed a one-term or one-year course. They might have a certificate, but they would not be eligible to be a full member of the major national association, the British Association for Counselling and Psychotherapy. This body has strict codes of conduct and guide-lines for members and would be able to tell you if the person you are thinking of seeing is indeed a current member.

Before you choose a therapy you should check out these facts by contacting the relevant association as well as asking the therapist. Other questions to ask include whether the therapist has insurance, for example. Professional associations are listed in the Appendix. By asking questions and checking up you should be able to avoid the charlatans as well as ensuring that you find a trained therapist.

What types of training do complementary therapists have to have?

Training for therapists ranges from short courses to diplomas or degrees. Many therapists are doctors, nurses, physiotherapists, radiographers or other health professionals who have undertaken extra training in a particular therapy. Some therapists will have only completed a recognised qualification in their specific field and others are teachers of techniques such as meditation and yoga based on ancient philosophies.

You should always check what qualifications a therapist has, whether they are registered with a national organisation or association (see previous question) and also what experience they have of working with people with cancer.

Are these complementary therapies expensive?

Not many therapies are available on the NHS and those that are may only be available in larger cancer centres. Many therapies involve a course of treatment lasting for several sessions and this could prove costly if you see a private therapist. Before you decide to embark on a course of treatment, you should ask exactly how many times you will be expected to attend, how often and how much it will cost.

Your breast care nurse may know of local – or national – support organisations which provide therapies in return for a small fee or donation, as mentioned in the introduction to this chapter.

Do complementary therapies take up much time?

Some do and some don't. Once you have learned how to use relaxation techniques you may find you can take a few minutes out relaxing whenever you like. On the other hand, counselling may require you to travel to the counsellor, have the session and travel back again, perhaps at a regular time each week for a number of weeks.

What if I don't have the willpower to keep using a particular therapy?

Many people worry that if they start to use a therapy they will have to continue for a long time, and some of the therapies mentioned in this chapter do require a lot of willpower. But if you don't want to carry on, for whatever reason, it is important that you stop, or you will be left feeling tied to something that started out as a matter of choice.

If I start a therapy and then give up, won't I feel I've failed and let everyone down?

Just as choosing to use a particular therapy should be your own decision, so stopping is up to you, too. It isn't a question of failing, rather it is a question of having tried something that isn't right for you or that has been useful but no longer feels that way. No one else has the right to tell you to continue when you don't want to.

Sometimes people stop using a therapy because it is too expensive or because they can no longer give the time necessary. It can be very hard to reach such a decision without feeling guilty about stopping, particularly if relatives or friends had been eager for you to take up the therapy in the first place. Yet, once again, the decision belongs to you and no one should attach blame or be angry about your choice.

ACUPUNCTURE

What is acupuncture?

Acupuncture is a treatment that has been practised for several thousand years. In China it is a standard form of medical treatment. The key principles behind it are:

- we all have a vital energy called Ch'i flowing throughout our bodies along pathways called meridians;

- if we are ill it is due to an imbalance in the body's Ch'i;

- this means that at least one of our 12 meridians is blocked – the Ch'i is not able to flow and so symptoms of disease appear in the parts of the body corresponding to the meridians;

- by inserting very fine special needles into certain points (acupoints) which lie along the meridians, energy can be diverted to areas where it is needed to treat the imbalance in Ch'i.

Can acupuncture be used to treat breast cancer?

No, but acupuncture is documented to relieve chronic pain, especially in combination with massage. Another form of acupuncture is electro-acupuncture, where a pulsating electrical current is applied to the acupuncture needles as a means of stimulating the acupoints; this was developed in China around 1934. Studies suggest that it may relieve sickness and fatigue arising from chemotherapy.

How many sessions of acupuncture would I need?

This is hard to say. How long treatment will last and how often you will need it to maintain any beneficial effects will vary from person to person. It will also depend on why you are having it and how long you have had the symptoms that you wish to treat.

Acupuncture to treat nausea and vomiting, for example, is given before each chemotherapy treatment begins. Acupuncture is often considered as an effective short-term treatment to bring immediate relief rather than a treatment with effects which last for months.

Do acupuncturists have to be specially trained?

Yes, they do. Some acupuncturists are medically qualified doctors, dentists, nurses or physiotherapists who have then been trained in acupuncture. Others may not have a medical background but have been trained as acupuncturists. It is one element of Traditional Chinese Medicine (see later).

Can I get acupuncture on the NHS?

Some acupuncturists do provide treatment on the NHS, working in hospitals or clinics.

ART THERAPY

What is art therapy?

Art therapy began in both England and America in the 1940s. It is now an established profession in many countries, with a recognised place in the process of healing. As part of the art therapy process, art materials (for example paints, clay and batik) are used to express your thoughts and feelings without words. A trained art therapist guides you in exploring the images you produce, helping you become aware of things you may not have realised or recognised. You can have art therapy on your own or in a group. Some people find drawing helpful even if they don't always share their work with an art therapist.

Do you have to be able to draw in the first place?

No, definitely not! Art therapy isn't about creating works of art: it's about using paper and paints or crayons to express yourself without having to find words.

Is art therapy useful for people who have breast cancer?

Yes, it can be useful, because it can help you to gain a greater understanding of yourself and of your cancer and treatment, as well as helping you to express your feelings.

How many art therapy sessions would I need?

That depends on you and your art therapist. Some people start to use art therapy when they are diagnosed with cancer and continue to use it throughout their treatment and beyond. Others may be introduced to it for the first time when they are terminally ill and may find it helps them to face dying.

Are art therapists specially trained?

Yes, there are training courses which people do in order to practise as art therapists. There are various approaches used in art therapy and the training differs for each of these. All of them will include some training in one or more psychological techniques so that you and your therapist can interpret your paintings or other images.

Can I get art therapy on the NHS?

Art therapy is sometimes available in cancer treatment centres and hospices; otherwise, it is a private treatment.

COUNSELLING

What is counselling?

Counselling is sometimes called a 'talking therapy'. A counsellor listens carefully to what you say about a particular situation. They then respond to you so you can explore and understand more clearly what you are feeling and thinking. It is private and confidential.

Counselling is no longer thought of as a complementary therapy but is included here as it is something you may choose to do for yourself.

I have plenty of people giving me advice! Why would I need counselling?

Counselling is not the same thing as giving advice. A counsellor does not direct you into a particular course of action or pass judgement on something you have said or done.

'If I were you I'd . . .' is giving advice. 'What do you think you might find helpful . . .? or 'How would you feel if . . .?' are examples of using a counselling approach, where any decisions are coming from you.

How can counselling help someone with breast cancer?

It can provide a space and a place to talk about your feelings, or about events current and past as well as hopes and fears. By offloading what is going round and round in your head, you may find you feel better able to cope and also get some useful strategies from the counsellor to help in feeling better in yourself.

Some examples of different styles of counselling are:

- **cognitive behavioural therapies** which focus on aspects of behaviour;

- **psychodynamic therapies** which are concerned with your past life and experiences; and

- **humanistic techniques** which concentrate on you as you are today taking into account some influences of the past.

Not every technique will suit everybody, so if you try one type of counselling and it doesn't feel right you might want to try another with a different counsellor.

How many sessions of counselling will I need?

The first time you go to see a counsellor you should end the session by both agreeing to a 'contract'. This covers the aim of your counselling sessions, and from this, how many times you plan to meet, how much each session will cost, how long sessions will last and where they will take place. This is not a legal agreement, even though it is called a contract: it's simply a word to describe whatever you and the counsellor have decided between you. You can, of course, change your 'contract' at any time, or stop your counselling sessions if you wish to do so.

Do counsellors have to be specially trained?

Yes, if they are to practise as counsellors they should have completed a professional training course. Counsellors or psychologists who wish to work with people who have breast cancer should have a recognised qualification or degree and be a member of one of the major associations for their professions (see Appendix). Ideally they should have some experience of working specifically with people who have cancer.

My practice nurse says she has counselling skills. Is this the same as being a counsellor?

Many people who provide support and a listening ear for people who have cancer have very good counselling skills but have not been professionally trained as counsellors. They are able to listen to what the person is saying and to respond in a caring and empathic way. They will not enter into a 'contract' of the sort described above and usually provide their services for free.

Can I get counselling on the NHS?

More and more cancer treatment centres employ counsellors who may be psychologists, nurses or therapy radiographers who have had additional training in counselling. Local cancer support and self-help groups may have counsellors in the group who will see people free of charge or for a small fee. Private counsellors will charge fees; some offer concessionary rates if you ask for them.

DIETS

Is there any special food I should eat because I have breast cancer?

No, there isn't one special diet to follow. Everyone, whether they have cancer or not, is advised to eat a healthy, well-balanced diet. For most people this means cutting down on the amount of fatty food they eat and having more fresh fruit and vegetables. This is a standard recommendation for general health, not a complementary therapy! Eating well is good for the people you live with too.

Why do some people decide to follow a new diet when they have breast cancer?

Following a new diet can lead some people to feel that they are helping themselves in a positive way. For some people a change in their diet can lead to a change in their attitude towards themselves. However, omitting certain food groups may actually reduce your body's immunity when you need it most so be wary of making any radical changes without first talking them through with your medical team.

What sort of diets are there for people with breast cancer?

There are many different diets that people might wish to try, and some of the better-known ones are mentioned here. It is worth noting that there is no peer-reviewed published clinical research to support the use of various diets for people with any type of cancer.

Always tell the hospital staff if you are planning to change your usual diet during the time you are having treatment, as some diets may make expected side effects of treatment (for example nausea) much worse. Hospital dietitians should be able to provide you with personal dietary advice during and immediately after treatment.

Some dietary therapies need lots of preparation and can be

expensive. This could have a big impact on any other people who live with you, as well as requiring you to follow an intensive regime, and you might wish to take this into account if you are choosing a diet.

Are supplements useful for helping to treat breast cancer?

You should be able to get enough nutrients from your food unless you have a deficiency or can't take in enough nutrients in the normal way. The use of supplements is an area of current research.

A friend mentioned the Bristol Diet. What is it?

This is a diet that was first used at the Bristol Cancer Help Centre (now **Penny Brohn Cancer Care** (address in Appendix). Each person is given individual attention to help them to use nutrition as a self-help tool. Its a wholefood diet, mostly vegetarian, with some animal protein as appropriate, or vegan.

Gerson Therapy involves a diet, doesn't it?

Yes, it does. Gerson Therapy views cancer as a chronic disease which upsets the body's metabolism. It is thought this can lead to tissue damage, especially in the liver, and to the immune system which governs the body's defences, making people more prone to infection and other illnesses. The therapy aims to help to make the body healthy by making the immune system function properly again.

The diet is one of fruit and vegetables that may be eaten raw, liquidised or steamed. Gerson Therapy involves using coffee or castor oil enemas to help to stimulate the liver to remove poisons from the body.

This diet claims to cure cancer but there is absolutely no evidence to support this.

What is the Macrobiotic Diet?

This diet is based on eating foods which complement each other in terms of **Yin** and **Yang**. Yin and Yang are two opposing but complementary principles in Chinese philosophy. Yin, which comes from the Chinese word for dark, represents feminine, dark and negative principles. Yang, which comes from the Chinese word for light, represents masculine, light and positive principles. Illness is attributed to an imbalance of these two principles.

Yin foods include fruit, and sweet, sour or hot foods, while Yang foods include cereals and foods of animal origin. By adapting your dietary balance of Yin and Yang foods to counteract the imbalance you may restore your health. Salt intake is strictly controlled and meat, milk and processed foods are not eaten at all in this diet.

Does eating dairy products cause breast cancer, or cause it to come back?

There have been claims that eating dairy products may cause breast cancer and also that avoiding them after diagnosis and treatment can make for a better outcome, but scientific research has been inconclusive in supporting this theory. A dairy-free diet, however, can limit your intake of calcium which is important for healthy bones, especially after the menopause.

Before changing your diet in this way, you should talk to your doctor, breast care nurse or a dietitian.

Many people are vegetarian, but what does this mean?

Vegetarians do not eat any meat or poultry, although some non-meat eaters do eat fish. Vegans also exclude all dairy products, eggs and such animal products as honey. If you decide to follow a vegetarian or vegan diet, it is important that you get enough protein and fatty acids.

HEALING

What is healing?

There are two types of healing: spiritual and psychic. Spiritual healing is the healing of the sick in mind, body and spirit. The healing is considered to come from divine energies through prayer and meditation. Psychic healing is similar but has no religious context.

The healer is a person who can harness healing energy, whatever its origin, and can then transfer this energy to the person being healed. It is thought that the transferred energy helps build up the energy field, or life force, of the person having healing, stimulating recovery from the disease or treatment.

A form of healing that has grown in popularity is Reiki (pronounced 'rake-ee'). This therapy claims to harness the body's own energy (rather than energy from outside) to help in healing. A number of complementary therapists with qualifications to practise other therapies (such as reflexology) are now following an additional training to practise Reiki.

Some studies have suggested that Reiki can reduce pain levels in people with cancer, while others have not found this to be the case.

Is it true that you don't actually have to be with a healer to have healing?

Yes, there are some healers who work at a distance, and so you are not required to visit them. Other healers prefer to make physical contact with the person being healed.

Can I get healing on the NHS?

Healing of either kind is not readily available on the NHS. Some healers do not charge a fee but might ask for a donation instead.

HERBAL MEDICINE

What is herbal medicine?

It is the use of herbs and plants to treat illnesses. Herbal remedies have been used since ancient times to treat a variety of disorders. It may be the roots, leaves, stem or seed that are used to make the preparation but they are used whole, unlike conventional drugs that just use the active ingredients. There are different types of herbal medicine, such as Western Herbal Medicine, Traditional Chinese Medicine and Ayurveda. You can get some herbs over the counter, or see a practitioner, who will prescribe a mixture specially suited to you.

Can herbal remedies be used to treat breast cancer?

There is no strong evidence to suggest that herbal remedies can be effective in treating breast cancer. Some conventional medicines come from plants, such as the vinca alkaloids used to treat leukaemia and other cancers but this is not the same as simply taking a herbal remedy for treatment.

Can I use herbal remedies to help with side effects of conventional treatment?

Some people find that nausea and vomiting from chemotherapy may be reduced by the use of some herbs. Others believe that fatigue may be relieved and the immune system may be supported. Herbal medicine may also help with menopausal symptoms caused by chemotherapy and hormone treatments, but do check with your specialist team.

If herbs are effective as medicine, does that mean they can also be dangerous?

Herbal remedies are classed as foodstuffs and are not controlled in the same way as medicines. This means that they do not need to be subjected to clinical trials and the preparations are not prepared to a given standard. Not all remedies are considered safe and some have been withdrawn because of concerns about effects on health or interactions with certain drugs. A qualified medical herbalist will know what may be helpful for you.

You should always discuss using herbal remedies with your doctor or breast care nurse before you start this therapy.

Do herbalists have to be trained?

Yes, there are degree courses for people who wish to become practitioners. Contact one of the professional associations listed in the Appendix.

Are herbal remedies available on the NHS?

No, they are not. You need to find a private practitioner and, to do this, you should contact a professional association to get the name of a qualified practitioner.

HOMEOPATHY

What is homeopathy?

It is a treatment involving the use of substances known as remedies. These are often added to small pills or pillules which you dissolve under your tongue or the remedy is given as a liquid of which you swallow one or two drops a day.

The word 'homeopathy' comes from two Greek words: *homo,*

similar, and *pathos*, suffering. The remedy that is prepared for you contains a very dilute amount of a substance which in larger quantities would produce similar symptoms to the illness that is being treated. In contrast, most modern medicine works on **allopathic** principles – 'allopathy' comes from the Greek words *allos*, other and *pathos*. Allopathic treatment has an effect on the body that is opposite to that caused by the disease.

Most remedies are derived from plants (such as belladonna or pulsatilla), and minerals (such as phosphorus and silica).

Do people use homeopathy to treat breast cancer?

Although not proven in clinical trials, some people choose to use homeopathic remedies alone. In practice no conventional doctors recommend homeopathy as an alternative treatment but may agree to it alongside conventional treatment.

How about using homeopathy for treating the side effects of treatment?

Some people find it helps reduce the effect of radiotherapy on their skin and relieves nausea and other side effects of chemotherapy. None of these benefits have been shown in clinical trials.

How does the homeopath decide on the correct remedy for me?

Your first consultation with a homeopath should last for at least an hour. During this time you will be asked questions about yourself and your lifestyle, about any physical symptoms you have and any medicine or treatment that has been prescribed for you. You will also be asked about the health of your close relatives both now and in the past. With all this information the homeopath will then select the remedy that most closely matches the symptom picture of the person, using their knowledge of the symptom pictures of all the remedies.

When this match is achieved the person's inner healing ability is thought to be activated and healing occurs.

Do homeopaths have special training?

Yes, they do. All homeopaths should have gained a recognised qualification in homeopathy before they practise.

Is homeopathy available on the NHS?

Yes it is, but not widely available. Your family doctor should be able to tell you if you can receive homeopathic treatment on the NHS in the area in which you live. There are homeopathic hospitals in London, Bristol and Glasgow.

HYPNOTHERAPY

What is hypnotherapy?

Hypnotherapy uses the technique of hypnosis to harness the power of your subconscious mind to help support you as you deal with your breast cancer and the treatments.

How could hypnosis help me?

Hypnosis may help you to cope with all the different emotions that a diagnosis of breast cancer brings. Additionally, a number of studies have suggested that hypnosis has a role to play before an operation in calming and relaxing people. After the operation it may aid healing, reduce pain, and reduce some of the side effects of chemotherapy such as nausea. Hypnotherapy may reduce the stress of chemotherapy, especially in people who hate needles, and radiotherapy or some scans if people feel claustrophobic.

Are hypnotherapists trained?

Yes, there are a number of training courses that people can take to become hypnotherapists.

Is there anyone who can teach me to use hypnosis on myself?

Certainly there is. Hypnotherapists can teach you self-hypnosis techniques to support you through your cancer journey. Hypnosis and visualisation (see below) often work closely together.

Is hypnotherapy available on the NHS?

Some cancer treatment centres may offer hypnotherapy alongside relaxation and visualisation.

MASSAGE

What exactly is massage, and what's it for?

Massage involves manipulation of the soft tissues, for example painful muscles, certain aches and stiffness, and it can help you to relax. It stimulates the circulation of blood and lymph round the body and this can encourage the removal of waste products and poisons.

Massage can be deep or gentle and the person who gives you the massage may work special oils into your skin which can enhance the effect of the massage. There are many different massage techniques which include kneading, pressing, rubbing, stroking and tapping. Shiatsu massage may be gentle or deep and can be deeply relaxing and can help relieve fatigue and other symptoms.

If I have massage, are there any types of massage I should avoid?

Massage for people with cancer only uses gentle, light massage movements. If you are thinking about a type of massage which involves vigorous rubbing or kneading or applying pressure to deeper parts of the body, discuss it first with your surgeon or breast care nurse.

Gentle massage, which can be very soothing and relaxing and can help you to feel good, is not likely to affect the cancer. For example, even a simple hand massage for about 10 minutes on each hand can be very relaxing.

Aromatherapy and reflexology are probably the two most frequently used professional techniques (see below). But a friend could give you a gentle massage at home, if they are careful to avoid the area where your cancer is or was.

I've heard that massage can be used to treat lymphoedema. What type of massage is this?

Lymphoedema is the swelling which can arise from a blockage of the lymph flow following surgery and radiotherapy. It can happen in the arm after treatment for breast cancer. Sometimes lymphoedema can be eased by two techniques: a type of massage called **manual lymph drainage** or MLD and special compression sleeves. This is a very specific type of massage and must only be given by a fully qualified practitioner. With thorough instruction, it can be done by yourself or a family member. Lymphoedema is discussed more fully in Chapter 5.

Is there special training for people who give massage?

Yes, some people may attend a two-day course and then decide to practise massage. However, professional associations now require massage therapists to have a diploma or degree before they can work with people with cancer. If you are going to seek out aromatherapy, reflexology or any other massage from a professional, check out their training and qualifications first, to make sure you get someone with suitable experience.

Is massage available on the NHS?

Generally speaking, no. Some health professionals may have taken courses in reflexology (massage on the feet or hands) and may practise it as part of their job. Aromatherapy is, however, gradually becoming more widely available in hospices and some cancer treatment centres.

What is aromatherapy?

Aromatherapy is a form of gentle massage treatment using extracts called essential oils which come from flowers, roots and leaves. The oils are diluted and massaged into the skin. The aromatherapist will make a blend of different oils specific for each individual person. Often the aromatherapist will play a relaxation tape while giving the massage to help you to relax.

How can aromatherapy help people who have cancer?

Combining the effects of gentle massage with the properties of the plant oils can make it an uplifting tonic for some people. For example, certain oils can help reduce swelling, others may help to strengthen the immune system and some can help you to relax. It is very important, however, that you don't have an aromatherapy massage on a part of the body where you are having, or have recently had, radiotherapy treatment as it might make the skin unnecessarily sore in that area. Several small studies have shown that this technique relieves anxiety in people who have cancer and may also help people to sleep better.

Could I use aromatherapy oils apart from as a massage?

Yes, you can and your aromatherapist may be able to recommend ways that can help you. Some oils can be diluted and added to bath water so that you can relax in the bath and gain benefit from the oils. This should only be done with guidance from a qualified aromatherapist. If you have recently had radiotherapy to certain parts of your body, you may have been advised not to have proper baths for a period of time. It is important to observe this and not bathe with oils until you are able to wash as usual.

You can buy burners for essential oils which release the oil vapours into the room when you use the burner. This can help you to relax and to combat certain side effects of treatment, such as nausea. Again ask for guidance as to what may be helpful for you.

What is reflexology?

It is a type of massage usually given to feet, although it can be given to hands. The whole body is seen as being mapped out on the feet – the right side of the body on the right foot and the left side on the left foot. The organs or tissues in a particular body zone are believed to be linked to reflex points on the feet (or hands) and massage of these points treats the corresponding part of the body. For example, the liver corresponds to a reflex point towards the outer side of the middle part of the sole of the right foot, and the spleen corresponds to a similar point on the sole of the left foot.

How does reflexology work?

There are different views as to how reflexology works. One view is that the gentle massage helps to improve blood circulation and stimulates the body's immune system. Another is that the body's natural energy flow is blocked by illness or stress and the reflexologist can feel a change in a particular reflex point which corresponds to the blocked part. Massage to this area can remove the blockage so that energy can flow freely again. A possible effect of reflexology is that the massage encourages the body to produce its own pain relief (endorphins) which could lead to fewer drugs being needed.

Can reflexology be useful for people who have cancer?

Yes, it can be for some people. Reflexology is not about curing an illness, rather it is focused on reducing stress and helping people to relax. When you are relaxed you are more likely to sleep better and be better able to cope with your cancer treatment and any side effects.

Can I practise reflexology at home?

Yes, you can. There are books that you can buy or get from the library that explain the principles of reflexology and how to use it. Perhaps you can learn with a friend so that you can give each other a reflexology massage. You should get advice from a qualified therapist before you do this.

How many sessions of aromatherapy or reflexology would I need?

That depends on why you are having it. For some people having just one session can be very beneficial, for others several sessions may be suggested by the therapist to achieve the desired effect.

MEDITATION

What is meditation?

It is a technique of using your mind in a way that aids relaxation and reduces stress and tension. Some types of meditation have a devotional or religious approach, others such as T'ai Chi have a physical approach. Meditation has been used for centuries and has been a part of both Eastern and Western cultures. Transcendental and mindfulness meditation are two commonly practised approaches. Transcendental meditation uses the repetition of a specific mantra to quieten the mind. Mindfulness is the practice of cultivating non-judgmental present moment awareness that can help relieve stress.

Meditation is not a useful technique for people who have borderline personality disorders or who have a history of psychotic illness.

Can meditation help someone who has breast cancer?

Yes, it can because meditating regularly can help to relieve anxiety and the symptoms of stress. It may lead to a person needing to take less pain relief, and the combination of all these things can result in an improved quality of life.

How do you learn to meditate?

You could start by reading a book and listening to a CD about meditation and trying out some of the basic concentration and breathing techniques. To study further you could go to a teacher experienced in the particular technique you wish to learn. Before learning to meditate you will have to learn relaxation techniques.

What happens the first time I go to a meditation teacher?

Well, that varies according to the type of meditation, but you should be told about the meditation and why it might be beneficial. You will then be taught the principles of meditation.

Do teachers have special training?

Many people who teach meditation are trained in mindfulness-based stress reduction or have been taught meditation techniques through other teaching, for example, Buddhism.

Is meditation teaching available on the NHS?

No, but some organisations that teach meditation do not charge.

NATUROPATHY

What is naturopathy?

The word 'naturopathy' is an umbrella term used to describe therapies from the mainstream areas of western natural medicine. These include nutrition (which includes diet and lifestyle modification and vitamin and mineral therapy), herbal medicine and homeopathy. Iridology, studying the iris of the eye, is often used as a diagnostic aid. Physical therapies may also be used, including therapeutic massage and remedial massage. (See the questions above for details about herbal medicine, homeopathy and massage.)

RELAXATION

What is relaxation?

Relaxation is a technique that can help to improve your quality of life by reducing tension, anxiety and fatigue. Relaxation involves becoming aware of all your muscles and of the tension in them, and then of gradually releasing that tension. Relaxation techniques can be learned either by attending classes or from a CD.

Can relaxation help people who have breast cancer?

Yes, it can be useful. For example, some people use relaxation techniques to help them to cope with chemotherapy and radiotherapy; others find they help them to sleep better after treatment.

Does the NHS provide relaxation teaching?

A number of cancer treatment centres have relaxation tapes or CDs for you to use. Some may also have a member of staff who can help you learn the techniques.

TRADITIONAL CHINESE MEDICINE

Traditional Chinese Medicine (TCM) is an ancient medical system that uses a deep understanding of the laws and patterns of nature and applies them to the human body. TCM has been practised for over 5,000 years.

TCM is holistic in its approach. A person's body, mind, spirit and emotions are seen as part of one complete circle rather than loosely connected pieces to be treated individually.

How does TCM help people with breast cancer?

A combination of acupuncture, Chinese herbs, exercises and diet will be suggested for you by a TCM practitioner. TCM philosophy believes that the body has the potential to heal itself or to slow down the progression of any disease.

Some herbal regimes may enhance the immune system, reduce the toxicity of chemotherapy and radiotherapy, improve symptoms and possibly act preventatively. There is little evidence from randomised clinical trials to support the efficacy of TCM, although it may help with nausea, tiredness and depression in women being treated for breast cancer.

Are TCM practitioners trained?

Yes they are. Some people may be qualified in one aspect of TCM but if they are qualified in all aspects they are registered with a national professional body.

Is TCM available on NHS?

Some TCM treatments, such as acupuncture, are available at larger cancer centres and some support centres.

VISUALISATION

What is visualisation?

Once you have learned relaxation techniques, you can learn to see an image in your mind and to alter it as you wish. This is visualisation.

How do I learn to visualise?

When you learn relaxation techniques you will be taught to picture a scene or an object as part of the relaxation process. Once you are able to create a particular image in this way, you will find you can create new images and make them act in any way you choose.

How can it be helpful for people who have breast cancer?

Many people find that if they can see their cancer in their mind they can visualise its destruction. For example, some people give their cancer a shape in their mind and imagine it being attacked or engulfed by something. Visualisation can also help some people to cope with the side effects of treatment. They might visualise something cool touching their skin where they have had radiotherapy treatment as a way of helping to soothe skin soreness that can occur as the course of treatment progresses.

Is visualisation available on the NHS?

Many cancer treatment centres who offer relaxation sessions also include visualisation techniques.

YOGA

What is yoga?

It is a health-giving practice which originated in India. When you practise yoga you learn breathing exercises combined with relaxation and holding certain positions. People who do regular yoga may find they feel better in their body and mind.

Can yoga help people who have breast cancer?

For some people it can be helpful because yoga can improve muscle and joint flexibility. However, it may not be suitable in all types of cancer, and you should check with your doctor and with the yoga teacher before starting to learn. Teachers should ask all pupils to fill in a medical questionnaire before they begin classes. The teacher can then adapt some of the work to make it more suitable for each person.

Are yoga teachers trained?

Yes, there are training courses for those wishing to teach yoga, although some people will run classes without having received any formal training. You should ask about a teacher's experience and also contact the national professional association to find someone who has worked with people who have cancer.

Can I practise yoga on my own once I have been taught?

Certainly you can carry out the exercises at home, but you should be very clear about what you can and can't do because of your cancer. Always check thoroughly with the teacher and possibly with the hospital doctor as well.

Can yoga be adapted to suit me if I can't move quite as before?

Yes, it can. There are books of exercises available that are written specifically for people who have chronic illnesses such as multiple sclerosis or who are in wheelchairs, and an experienced teacher should be able to guide you as well.

5 | Immediately after treatment

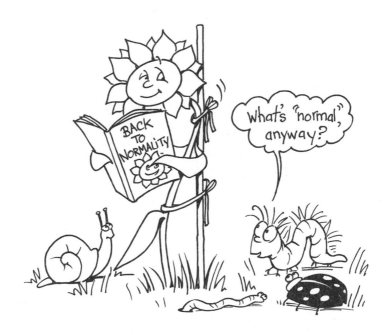

Many people feel quite unsettled after their breast cancer treatment is complete. Some may still be experiencing side effects and many will worry that the treatment might not have worked and that the breast cancer will come back.

Everyone recovers at their own pace, and therefore some of the issues discussed here, such as going back to work, will be early priorities for some people, while for others they will not become important until much later. Because of this, we deal with several topics both in this chapter and in the following one, which talks about living with cancer in the longer term. If the answers given here are brief, more detailed information will be found in Chapter 6 and vice versa.

TREATMENT

Will I feel better immediately after treatment?

You may feel that your health has improved in the weeks following treatment but sometimes it takes longer to recover from the effects of therapy itself. You may continue on treatment for five years if you are taking hormone therapy. There may also be later effects of treatment that make you feel you are not getting better as quickly as you would like.

Progress is often gradual. You can't recover overnight from a major operation or a course of intensive radiotherapy or chemotherapy. Some days you may think you are back to normal while on others you may feel depressed and tired. This is not unusual.

Will I have to go back to hospital for check-ups?

Yes. You may be seen a bit more frequently at first while you recover from your treatment but after this you may only need to visit once or twice a year. This routine follow-up will be an outpatient appointment, during which the doctor or nurse can examine you, check if you have any new symptoms or problems and observe how you are and how you are adapting to life after your treatment. You are unlikely to need regular tests except a mammogram every one to two years but you may have other tests if you develop a new symptom that needs investigating.

Many people feel anxious when their follow-up appointment is getting close. It is natural to worry about what might be found and you might find it helpful to talk to the staff at the hospital or to someone from a cancer support group or organisation (see Appendix) about how you are feeling.

Will I be able to stop going back for check-ups?

This is quite likely. Many people are discharged from attending outpatient appointments after a few years of follow-up, although you will still need to have mammograms. If you have been discharged, your GP can always refer you back to your hospital team if any new symptoms appear, or you can contact your breast care nurse directly.

While I was going to hospital regularly for treatment, I had hospital transport provided. Can I continue with this?

Possibly. You should talk to your doctor about it. An ambulance or hospital car is only provided if it is necessary on medical grounds. You may find that once treatment is completed and you start to feel better, you can make your own way to and from the hospital by public transport or by driving yourself.

I feel well enough to travel to the hospital but the fares are quite expensive. Can I get any help with them?

Yes, you may be able to get help with your fares. You can visit your local benefits office for advice, or contact your breast care nurse. **Macmillan Cancer Support** can also advise you regarding fares, a refund of parking fees or, in London, the congestion charge. You can find their details in the Appendix.

If I need a new breast prosthesis, do I have to pay?

Probably not. Each prosthesis has a guarantee, usually for two to three years so you can get it replaced after normal wear and tear and sooner if you accidentally damage it (providing this does not happen too often). You may also be re-fitted for a new product if your shape or weight change and your existing prosthesis no longer fits you. If you have been discharged from routine follow-up appointments, your GP may need to refer you back to the hospital to get your replacement.

If I am continuing to take hormone therapy for five years do I have to pay prescription charges each time?

Not necessarily; it depends on whether or not you receive any benefits. Discuss this with your doctor or the pharmacy staff. You may be eligible for exemption from prescription charges or you may benefit from buying a pre-paid prescription card as this can save money over the long term.

RECURRENCE

What should I look out for which may indicate my cancer has come back?

It is difficult to list every symptom to look for, and many of these could occur for lots of reasons other than the cancer coming back. Generally, you should report any noticeable changes in your health, or anything which is unusual for you, that persists over several weeks without getting better and which does not have an obvious cause. Not every ache, pain, lump or change will mean that your cancer has returned, although this may be the first thought that comes to mind. However, report any new signs or symptoms to your doctor. If the problem is unrelated to your cancer, your mind will be put at rest and if it is a sign of a recurrence, treatment can be given.

Is there anything I can do to stop my cancer coming back?

There is nothing guaranteed. Some research studies have shown that people who take regular exercise have a better outlook after their breast cancer. This can be difficult after the onslaught of all your treatment but many people feel they want to make some changes to their lifestyle to improve general health and well-being. Don't put too much pressure on yourself but try to build up to taking regular exercise to improve your overall health.

DEALING WITH CHANGE

The doctors say my operation was a success and everyone is pleased with my progress but I can't look at my scar without flinching and I can't accept the changes in my body. Is this normal? How long will it take to adjust?

Your reaction is both normal and natural. Most people go through a period of adjustment to change and the time this takes varies from person to person. It often helps to talk about how you are feeling – with your partner, family and friends or one of the staff caring for you. There are many people you can turn to for practical and emotional support. Choose someone with whom you feel comfortable – your hospital doctor, your family doctor, a specialist nurse or someone else you became close to at the hospital. This help and support can be extended to your family if they too are finding it difficult to adjust to what has happened to you. Some hospitals employ trained counsellors with whom you can discuss your feelings and concerns about various aspects of your life.

You can also turn to someone from a cancer support group or organisation such as those listed in the Appendix. There are many breast cancer specific support groups where you can meet others who have been through something similar. It can feel very supportive to be among people who have probably felt similar to the way you do now.

I seem to have lost my confidence. When I go out I'm sure everyone knows I've had breast cancer and I'm different. Is there anything I can do to overcome this?

Many people feel less confident about meeting others, especially if you now look different. It takes time to regain your confidence in the same way as it takes time for you to adjust to the changes caused by treatment for cancer. Very often, adjustment and self-confidence go hand in hand.

If you are in company, the only person who may know of or notice any difference may be you. Friends, colleagues or strangers will only know if you choose to tell them.

You may find it helpful to make contact with a person who has had the same operation or treatment as you. This is possible through many of the support and self-help organisations listed in the Appendix.

Everyone keeps telling me to put it all behind me, but it is really difficult. Am I being pathetic?

Having breast cancer and the treatment for it is like being on a huge emotional rollercoaster. Once treatment is over, the rest of the world expects you to 'get back to normal'. Sometimes you just aren't physically up to it because the impact of treatment can last some weeks and occasionally months. And you may still be taking hormone therapy that reminds you of your cancer and all you have been through. So while you still feel less than a hundred per cent others around you are only too delighted that you have come through the treatment. Often, because of their own fears as much as anything else, they want to see you as you were before it all happened. However, the old 'normal' may not be possible to achieve after the challenges you have faced.

Don't be pressured by others into doing things you don't want to do. Take time to consider decisions and don't hesitate to seek support of a counsellor to help you to adapt to life now that treatment is over.

PRACTICAL MATTERS

Can I drink alcohol now my treatment is over?

Yes, and in fact you may have been told you could have a drink during treatment if you wished. There is no reason why you shouldn't have a drink, but avoid having too much alcohol for the good of your general health.

Is it OK to go swimming after treatment?

Yes, although until your skin has healed from radiotherapy, it will remain sensitive and your doctor may advise against it just in the short term, in case chlorine in a pool irritates the area. Once everything is healed, it is safe to swim.

If you have had a mastectomy, you may feel less confident about going swimming. Your breast care nurse can offer advice on how to adapt swimming costumes and where to buy special swimwear. You can also get information about this from organisations such as **Breast Cancer Care** (see Appendix).

After my operation I was given special exercises to do by the physiotherapist. How long do I need to continue these?

Check with your breast care nurse or **physiotherapist** when to stop any special exercises. These will have been given to you to help you heal and to increase your range of movement. You need to carry on with them for the right length of time or you may not gain the full benefit from them and problems, such as stiffness, may occur later. Some people choose to carry on doing the exercises for years because they have got into a routine and it helps reassure them that they are reducing the chances of any arm problems in the future.

I haven't been able to do very much around the house. When can I begin doing shopping and housework?

Generally, whenever you feel able to. Housework is a more energetic activity than we tend to think so start slowly with dusting, washing-up and cooking light meals. Gradually add in other activities such as vacuuming, ironing and going out shopping. Remember your strength and range of movement will be less on the side of the surgery and you may well have lower energy levels after treatment. You will usually be given specific advice by the doctor or physiotherapist about what you can and cannot do in the weeks after surgery. In most cases, very energetic activities and heavy lifting are best avoided for a few weeks but don't worry if it takes longer before you feel back to normal. Everyone recovers at their own pace.

I can't wait to get out in the garden. Is gardening a good kind of exercise?

Yes, and it gets you out into the fresh air. However, you should start with light jobs like weeding and not try to dig the vegetable patch or mow the lawn in one go. And remember to take care to avoid cuts and infections if you have had surgery to your lymph nodes under the arm because of the risk of developing lymphoedema. Wear gloves when you garden and wash any cuts and apply an antiseptic cream.

The nurse mentioned lympheodema. What is it exactly?

Lymph is a colourless liquid that is formed by the tissues of the body. It is normally taken back into the bloodstream through the small tubes and glands which make up the lymphatic system. Lymphoedema occurs when this liquid builds up in the tissues under the skin. It causes swelling (oedema) in a limb or another part of the body. The tubes and glands of the lymphatic system may be damaged by treatment for cancer and so the lymph can't drain away, resulting in swelling.

Can I do anything to prevent getting lymphoedema?

It is not usually possible to prevent lymphoedema. However, your doctor can tell you if there is a chance that you may develop it because of the type of surgery or radiotherapy you have had. The doctor, physiotherapist and nursing staff can suggest ways to reduce the likelihood of developing lymphoedema.

- Use your 'at risk' arm normally. Gentle non-repetitive exercise, such as swimming, will keep your joints supple and assist lymph drainage.

- Don't use your arm for sudden or strenuous movements like pushing objects or carrying heavy shopping or a heavy shoulder bag on this side.

- Take care of your skin – wear gloves when gardening or doing housework, as an infection in a cut or scratch can trigger a swelling. Use an insect repellent to reduce the risk of bites or stings.

- Don't have blood taken from, or injections given into, the treated side. Ask the doctors or nurses to use your other arm. If you have had both sides treated, it is best to alternate sides.

- Don't wear tight clothing, like tight-fitting bras or sleeves that can cause constriction, or have your blood pressure measured on the treated side.

More information can be obtained from several organisations listed in the Appendix, such as the Lymphoedema Support Network.

If I get lymphoedema, can it be treated?

Yes. More is now known about why lymphoedema develops and how it can be treated. Several methods are used to control swelling including special massage techniques called manual lymph drainage (MLD) and elastic support sleeves. Treatment will be more effective if it is started as soon as you notice any swelling. Even if swelling is mild or comes and goes, report it to your doctor.

During my treatment I have put on a lot of weight. Will I get back to my normal weight again?

It is possible to lose the extra weight but it will take time. Try to set yourself realistic goals and plan to take regular exercise, for example, a daily walk. You can ask a dietitian at the hospital or your GP for advice about a healthy eating plan.

I am getting some pretty terrible menopause-like effects. Are these because of the hormone therapy?

If you were still having periods before you had chemotherapy, and your periods have stopped as a result – either temporarily or permanently – then this could be causing these symptoms. Hormone therapies can also cause side effects like menopausal symptoms. These can include hot flushes, night sweats, vaginal dryness, dry skin and hair, mood changes and difficulty concentrating.

Will the menopausal problems get better over time?

Yes, they should do. Most women notice they get better over a few months, whatever the cause. However, some find they don't improve and on rare occasions decide not to continue with their hormone treatment because of the side effects.

There are ways of minimising menopausal symptoms without drugs and you could contact organisations such as the **Women's Health Concern**, listed in the Appendix, for suggestions about these, which include diet, vaginal lubricants and complementary therapies.

Sometimes I sit down to read a book or write a letter and find I can't concentrate. Is this normal after treatment?

Lack of concentration is not uncommon. It may be due to the effects of treatment or simply because you have not fully adjusted to having had a serious illness. Usually when we are ill, even if it's just a bout of flu, we feel mentally less alert and less able to concentrate. Studies have shown that chemotherapy can result in poor concentration and memory and this can take many months to improve. If you don't feel you are recovering as quickly as you should, it may be useful to talk to someone about this. It may help to set your mind at rest that you are not unusual.

How soon after treatment can I start driving again?

You should discuss this with your doctor. Your physical movements may be restricted or a seat belt may cause discomfort to your chest after surgery. However, you can usually drive about four to six weeks after your operation. If you drive when your doctor has advised you not to, your insurance may be invalid if you have an accident.

I feel pretty well, all things considered. Is there anything I shouldn't do?

Not really, but check with your doctor if you are in any doubt. Occasionally, a person will be given specific advice which may only need to be followed for a short time or which may be relevant in the longer term. For example, if you have had chemotherapy, or any other treatment which has affected your blood count, you may be advised to avoid crowded places for a while immediately after treatment because you might still be at risk of picking up an infection more easily. But this sort of advice will only need to be followed in the short term.

When will I feel able to get out and about more with my friends and family?

Whenever you feel ready to do so. The time you choose will depend on how you feel physically, how confident you are about mixing with other people and what you want to do. The important thing is not to overtire yourself by doing too much too soon.

I don't have the energy to go out with friends or do the things I did before treatment. I don't feel I'm achieving anything. What can I do?

Any illness unsettles your normal routine and if you are used to being busy it is very frustrating when you don't feel able to take part in your usual activities. Recovery, both physical and emotional, is gradual. You may have up days and down days. Try to take advantage of the days when you have more energy and have a few activities lined up in preparation for such a day. Even if you don't feel like going out, family and friends can visit or you might like to take up a new hobby, something you always wanted to do but never had time for before.

Fatigue after treatment for breast cancer is very common so you may feel reassured to know you are not alone and that reduced energy levels are very unlikely to be related to the cancer coming back. **Cancerbackup** publish a booklet, *Coping with Fatigue*, which you may find helpful (see Appendix for contact details).

I really miss my job. When can I go back to work?

This will depend to a large extent what your job entails. You may have continued working, full-time or part-time, during your treatment. If you were unable to work, discuss the possibility of returning on a part-time basis with your employer. If you have been working part-time during treatment you may be able to go back full-time quite soon.

If your job is mentally stressful or involves heavy manual work you may need a longer interval between finishing therapy and returning to work.

Depending on how you feel, you might wish to discuss this with your doctor, the occupational health department at your work or your employer to help you come to a decision.

What I really need is a break. Is there any reason why I can't go on holiday?

No, it's a good idea to plan a holiday or short break as soon as you feel well enough but you may have to take some extra factors into consideration. For example, you may need to check you have enough medicine for the time you are away. If you have only just finished treatment you may need to take a doctor's letter containing details of your illness, in case you need care while on holiday.

Sometimes holiday insurance may be more expensive after treatment for breast cancer, so you may have to shop around. Some of the organisations listed in the Appendix will be able to provide you with more information.

We are taking this opportunity to have a good holiday. Is it all right to go sunbathing?

As a general rule anyone who sunbathes should protect exposed skin with a sunblock cream and wear a hat and avoid the hottest time of the day. If you have had radiotherapy, the part of the body that was treated should be protected as the skin will be more sensitive. Some chemotherapy agents, for example 5fluorouracil and methotrexate, can also make your skin more sensitive and may cause an unusual darkening of the skin. If you have had these drugs you should be particularly careful to avoid bright sunlight.

Check with your doctor and follow all the rules about protecting your skin from the sun.

How soon can I resume sexual activity?

This varies from individual to individual and it is up to you to decide when, and if, you wish to start having sex again.

If you have lost interest in sex during your illness and treatment, you will probably find your feelings return once you are well again and have got used to the physical and emotional changes caused by your treatment. You may find sexual activity more tiring or difficult at first, but this will improve with time.

You may find that changes in the way your body looks and feels make you worry about loss of attractiveness, femininity or masculinity. Talking to your partner about these feelings may help to dispel them. You may wish to discuss your thoughts and fears with others, such as a specialist nurse or a counsellor. Don't be embarrassed about this; it is an important aspect of your recovery and adjustment.

Practical problems may result from your treatment, for example, chemotherapy causing an early menopause or side effects of hormone treatments may mean you have vaginal dryness which can make sexual intercourse uncomfortable. You may wish to try some of the range of vaginal lubricants available from the chemist.

Patience may be required and your sexual relationship may resume slowly. There are many ways of meaningful love-making and pleasurable sexual contact. You may find that this is the time to explore them.

MAKING CONTACTS

Now all my treatment is finished and I'm not going back to the hospital so often, I feel really alone. Who can I talk to?

Even though you are no longer attending hospital, it doesn't mean you can't get in touch with the staff there. If you have concerns of a medical nature, you should contact your GP or breast care nurse as soon as possible so that you don't worry unnecessarily. Your breast care nurse can also be contacted to discuss practical and emotional problems. She will probably encourage you to telephone if you are feeling low or have questions about what is happening. If you wish to take advantage of this offer, then do so – they really do mean what they say.

You may find you are more comfortable talking with your family doctor whom you may have known for a long time and who also knows your family well. Some practices also have specialist community nurses or counsellors attached to them, who may be able to help and support you.

How can I find someone who really understands how I feel?

There are many people who have been through a similar experience of breast cancer and treatment, who will identify with you. There are several voluntary organisations which might be able to help you, some of which were originally set up by people with cancer or their families, and are now national charities. There are other groups of people with a common interest in a particular aspect of health or illness. Details of these organisations are given in the Appendix. Some of them offer a confidential telephone service, providing information and support. Others can give you a list of local support and self-help groups, if you wish to meet with people in your own area, or they may have a network of people throughout the country who you can talk with or meet individually.

What's the difference between a support group and a self-help group?

It's probably easier to think first of the similarities rather than the differences. In fact the two terms are often interchangeable. Both are places where people can go to meet others who are going through, or have been through, similar experiences. Self-help groups, however, are generally only for the person who has had cancer, whereas support groups may be open to anyone affected by cancer in any way, including friends and relatives. Some groups may be run by professionals, for example breast care nurses, and some by people who have had cancer themselves.

I don't want to sit around listening to everyone describing what happened to them. Isn't this what happens in a support group?

No. People go to groups for lots of different reasons. Often the most important one is to meet people who have been through a similar experience to themselves. Being amongst people who can really identify with you and your experience can be very strengthening and positive. In such company many people feel they can relax and that they don't have to be concerned about putting on a brave face as they might have to for their friends or family.

Support groups usually offer a variety of activities which may include:

- regular meetings with an invited speaker followed by time to chat;

- regular 'drop-in' times for people to get together with no formal structure;

- the opportunity to try certain complementary therapies;

- counselling or befriending;

- social events.

There are also support networks where you might get telephone or internet support from someone in the same situation as you, but who you may never meet face to face.

For many people, being part of a cancer support group or network helps them to adjust to living with cancer. For information about organisations that can help you find support turn to the Appendix.

6 | Life with and after breast cancer

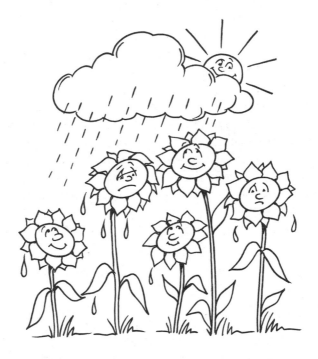

Having breast cancer is probably going to affect the way you lead your life, both during and after treatment. You may feel a wide range of emotions when you are told you have cancer and when you are going through treatment. The reactions of people close to you, such as friends or relatives, may also affect you.

There may be aspects of your life you decide to alter as a result of having breast cancer. Some things you may have to change, and for these you need to make some adjustments.

Practical, emotional and psychological support are all available for someone who has breast cancer, as well as for friends, partners and other relatives, although not everyone needs this. The Appendix describes the information and support organisations and the services they provide.

TALKING ABOUT BREAST CANCER

How can I find someone to talk to who has been through something similar?

There are several ways you can find support or share your experiences, feelings, hopes and fears with people who may have been in a similar situation.

- By making contact with a local breast cancer support or self-help group. Many areas have these and your breast care nurse can provide you with details of what is in your area. Some groups are only for the person who has breast cancer but many will include relatives and friends too, and there are special support groups for younger women with breast cancer. Some groups are for women with secondary breast cancer. Group activities vary from regular meetings, perhaps with a speaker, to social events. How often a group meets and the time of day varies from group to group. Regular telephone support groups, that enable people to be in touch without having to travel, are run by Breast Cancer Care (see Appendix).

- By speaking to someone on the telephone. There are organisations that provide information over the phone about breast cancer and its treatment. They have trained staff who can give you the time and space to talk, as well as trying to help you to find answers to any questions. They can also help you to work out the questions you would like to ask your doctor, for example. If you choose to telephone such an organisation you don't have to give your name. Some organisations will call you back to save you the cost of a long phone call; others operate a freephone system.

Some services also provide support by email. Most of these services will employ the same staff as the telephone staff to answer your questions. There may be a delay of a few days before you get a reply.

Increasingly organisations are exploring the use of on-line discussion boards or 'live' Internet talk. This does not mean you join a group unless it is a closed group and you all agree to participate; rather it is another way of receiving one-to-one immediate support and information through typing rather than talking.

- By surfing the Internet. You will find thousands of different options here. It is really important that you carefully check who is putting out the information. If it is a person who does not have a recognised qualification in cancer care but has their own experience to share, you should be aware that there is no medical back-up for the site and that what you are sharing are personal and not professionally endorsed opinions.

- By asking at the hospital where you go for treatment. Some hospitals know of local people who have been treated there or who attend clinics for check-ups, and who are willing to come in and talk with you.

- By speaking to someone who has had breast cancer. Some organisations offer 'peer support' – they train women, and men, who have had different types of breast cancer and who are of different ages, to offer support to other women and men who are going through a similar diagnosis or experience. This is not counselling or a formal relationship, more a supportive time you can spend either face-to-face or on the phone with someone who has been down a similar path to the one you are now on.

- By going to a cancer help centre. Increasingly, there are places that offer 'retreats' for people affected by cancer where you stay for a few days or a weekend. You could find out about these on the Internet or perhaps from your cancer treatment centre. Do check out carefully what they offer as some offer activities such as yoga and gentle massage while others offer cleansing diets and '**detoxification**' methods. While the former may be fine for you, the latter kind might not be helpful depending on your treatment, progress through the treatment plan, side effects you have or might have and so on. It is always advisable to check with your oncologist before embarking on a retreat programme. Most places that offer retreats charge for their services so check the cost first. Some may offer reduced rates in certain circumstances.

I've got breast cancer. Should I talk about what is happening or not?

That is for you to decide. Some people choose right at the start to talk openly and honestly to their partner, other relatives or close friends or work colleagues. Through this they are able to share the feelings they experience and can gain support and strength to cope with what is happening. Other people prefer not to talk about what is going on. They may cope well with what is happening but sometimes it can be hard for others to deal with their silence. Partners, relatives and friends will have their own feelings about what is happening to you and how it affects them, and problems with communication can arise if your breast cancer becomes a taboo subject that must not be mentioned.

I want to talk about things but it's hard to know where to start. What if I cry and can't stop?

Many people think that if they allow themselves to cry in front of someone else they will cause greater distress to themselves and to the other person. While it can be very painful to let yourself cry 'in public' it can be very beneficial in the end. Bottling up feelings means they will probably force their way out sooner or later and in a way that might be less within your control. Having breast cancer is an extremely emotional experience but sharing those feelings, rather than keeping them all inside, can relieve some of the tension. It may help you to face whatever lies ahead with support and understanding from people who are important to you.

Some people say they are frightened to cry in case they can't stop. No one cries constantly and there are no rules about when it is OK to cry and when it is not, although in some cultures some types of emotional expression are less acceptable than others.

Some people say they cry alone and that feels right for them.

It can also help you if you write down some of the thoughts in your head at the time. Writing like this is another way of releasing tension and of helping you to name what you are fearful of and sad about. This in turn can help you recognise if you would like some help to cope better, or maybe to find specific ways of dealing with particular problems. Some people like to keep what they have written in the form of a journal or diary, while others may tear it up and throw it away.

It is at this time that some people contact a breast cancer support and information organisation. Talking in private on the phone to a person you don't know and aren't likely to meet gives you the chance to practise what you might want to say to friends or relatives. This can make it easier when you do talk with them.

I am 48 and have just been told I have breast cancer. What should I tell my children?

Children are likely to notice if you are not quite your usual self, and may feel they are in some way to blame if they are not given any sort of explanation. Exactly what you tell them will probably depend on their ages, but as a general rule it is likely to be better for the whole household in the long run if you can tell them as much of the truth as possible. You may wish to tell it to them gradually over a period of time, or you may tell an older child more in the first instance than a younger child, although the older child may then tell the younger one anyway. If you are going to have treatment that could make you poorly, or if you are going to be in hospital, you may also find it helpful to tell your children's teachers, so that they are aware and can help to support the child in their class.

I am in for some lengthy treatment. What should we tell the school?

It can be really helpful for the children if their teachers are told exactly what is going on. Sometimes children use school as a place where they don't have to think about cancer and what is going on at home. No one would ever know that anything was happening. Other children act out their anxiety at school and their behaviour may change. If teachers know what is happening at home they can support the children as needed and this can relieve pressure on the whole family.

How much should the children know about what is going on with my breast cancer treatment?

This really depends on the age of the children (see previous questions). One of the most important things for a young child is that they feel that everything continues as normal and that their lives are the same as before. To help achieve this, it is important to maintain their routine as far as possible. Perhaps other mums at school or day care could help by picking up your children, for example, to give you some quiet time, especially if you are having daily radiotherapy or are in the middle of a course of chemotherapy.

Should I tell my teenage children what is going on with my breast cancer?

Teenage children, particularly girls, may be worried not only about their mum or dad with breast cancer but for themselves too. They may need some special time alone with you where you do some mother/father and daughter activity that gives them the time and opportunity to talk if they wish to. It can help if their closest friends' parents know what is happening in case their teenagers raise the subject.

Whilst many teens won't talk even if asked, they will certainly talk with their friends, perhaps using Internet chatrooms or phone calls.

I am worried about the impact my illness is having on the children. Is there any help for them?

There are organisations that offer information for families and teachers and produce booklets and information sheets. Some also provide support groups by telephone or Internet for children, including teenagers, whose parents have cancer (see Appendix).

If I have breast cancer, how do I know if my daughters are likely to get it?

The vast majority of breast cancers happen by chance and only a very small number of cases (less than 10%) are genetic and may run in families. Whether your daughters are at any increased risk will depend on how old you were when you developed breast cancer and whether there are any other close family members affected as well. Even if you do carry a faulty gene, you won't necessarily pass it on to your children, who would only have a 50:50 chance of inheriting it. If your daughters are at an increased risk, there are things that can be done, such as screening them from an earlier age, for example using MRI scans. For more details of the process of genetic screening, see Chapter 1.

PRACTICAL HELP

I've always been a person who gives help, not asks for it. Now I have breast cancer, how do I ask for help?

Look at this the other way round. Relatives and friends often find it hard to know where to start to help someone who is having treatment for breast cancer, or recovering from treatment. Asking for support means that people can feel useful and helpful, and you don't have to try to be superhuman to cope with everyday life on top of treatment. People do like to help.

Initially you could ask for help with practical things like picking up your children from school, helping to do your shopping, cooking a meal for you, or you could ask for company when you have hospital appointments. Then as time goes on and people offer their help, do take it or ask them if they would mind doing something else instead if there is a task you need doing.

DIET

Do I need to be careful about what I eat now I am having treatment?

It is sensible to eat a well-balanced diet because it is better for your general health. For most of us, eating a better balanced diet means having less fatty food, cutting down on our salt intake and eating more fibre in the form of fresh vegetables and cereals. Eating this type of diet is good for everyone, not just for people who have had breast cancer. A balanced diet will make sure that you get the vitamins and minerals you need to help your body to recover from any treatment you have had and to build you up again.

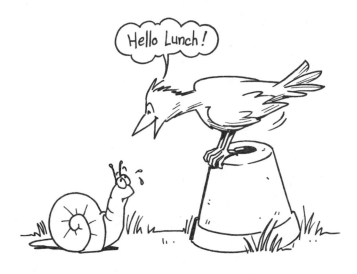

Do I need a special diet now I know I have breast cancer?

Some people choose to follow a particular complementary diet when they have breast cancer and continue with this after their hospital treatment ends. If you wish to try a new eating plan which is very different from your usual diet, make sure you let the hospital doctor know what you are planning. This is because some diets could make certain side effects of treatment, such as diarrhoea, rather worse or last longer. It might be better to wait until these are over before changing to a new style of eating. Information about some specific complementary diets can be found in Chapter 4.

Will changing my diet help to prevent my cancer from coming back?

There is no research which suggests that changing your diet would do this. Some people claim certain diets have helped to cure their breast cancer but there is no convincing evidence to support these claims. Do speak to your doctors about any diets you are considering because some of them can affect other parts of the body. For example, after the menopause women's bones become thinner and they are at a higher risk of osteoporosis (thinning of the bones) so a diet without calcium can be harmful to bones.

DRINKING ALCOHOL

What about drinking alcohol if you have breast cancer?

You should avoid having too much alcohol as it is not good for your general health. An occasional short, glass of wine or a beer is unlikely to be harmful. UK guidelines suggest women should not drink more than two units of alcohol a day (one unit is a small glass of wine, a single measure of spirits or half a pint of beer or cider). For men the maximum is three units daily. Table 1 (overleaf) gives more information.

SMOKING

I've got breast cancer. Should I stop smoking?

Whilst the strict medical answer to this is going to be 'yes', it is not quite that simple. If you have breast cancer, then you may want to adopt a new approach to life in general which could include giving up smoking. But while it is clear that smoking is a major cause of lung cancer and heart disease, there is no evidence that it causes breast cancer or will affect the chances of your breast cancer coming back. As well as this the stress of giving up on top of the stress of coping with a diagnosis and treatment can make it a big extra burden you might not feel you can face just now – and if you don't succeed, you may feel even worse. Some people find that while having chemotherapy they go off smoking anyway.

If you need help to give up, talk to your GP.

Table 1 Alcoholic drinks and units

Drink	Serving size	Units of alcohol
Spirits, e.g. whisky, vodka, rum, gin	25 mL	1
Spirits, e.g. whisky, vodka, rum, gin	35 mL	1.5
Lager, 3.5–4.5% vol (e.g. Tennent's, Fosters)	pint	2.2
Lager, premium, Special Brew	pint	4.5
Lager, alcohol free, bottled	300 mL	Trace
Beer (bitter)	pint	2.2
Stout, Guinness	pint	2.4
Cider, dry	pint	2.7
Cider, sweet	pint	2.7
Wine, dry white or red, 12.5% vol	125 mL	1.6
Wine, dry white or red, 12.5% vol	175 mL	2.2
Wine, med. white, 12.5% vol	125 mL	1.6
Wine, sparkling, 10% vol	125 mL	1.2
Sherry, dry, 20% vol	50 mL	1
Sherry, med. 20 % vol	50 mL	1
Port	50 mL	1

EXERCISE

Should I be taking exercise during treatment and after it has finished?

Exercise is good to stimulate the heart and to tone up flabby muscle, but if you are not used to exercising regularly, you should be careful. Don't start to do too much too soon, either during your treatment or afterwards, as you do not want to tire yourself out. Gentle, regular exercise throughout your treatment and beyond is far better for your body than sudden, strenuous activity when treatment is over.

If you are used to doing regular exercise, gym workouts or playing team sports, you may need to reduce what you do while having treatment and then increase slowly as side effects ease. It is a good idea to take advice from your oncologist, breast care nurse or a fitness professional about this.

Research is suggesting that taking exercise after breast cancer may improve the chances of it not coming back, so this is another reason why regular exercise is a good idea.

I am nearly finished with my treatment. Are there any forms of exercise which are better than others for me to take up now?

It is well known that swimming is a good way of exercising your whole body. However, you should avoid swimming if, for example, you have recently completed a course of radiotherapy – your skin will be sensitive on the part of your body that was treated, and chlorine could make any skin reaction to treatment worse. Some gym activities might be good to help you build up muscle tone again but you should try to find a balance between this type of exercise and pushing yourself too hard.

In general, if you are used to doing one particular type of exercise, then you may wish to continue with it. However, you might need to modify how much you do to take account of the fact that your body is not quite back to its usual state. Check with your doctor or breast care nurse before doing any exercise that involves heavy lifting or shoulder movements on the side of your axillary surgery.

THE SUN

Can I sit out in the sun after I've had breast cancer?

Yes you can, but do be careful. If you have had radiotherapy, the area treated will be much more sensitive to sun and you can easily burn. Use a high factor sunblock and keep the areas where you had treatment covered during the hottest times of the day.

Can I swim in the sea or a pool if it is sunny?

If you are swimming when there is strong sunlight, you should put on a waterproof sunblock and then cover up any treated area if possible. For example, you could wear a T-shirt. Better still, avoid the strongest sunlight. Remember to take care even if it is cloudy, as the sun's rays still filter through.

HOLIDAYS

Can I go on holiday straight after having treatment?

Usually, yes. It can be very beneficial to get away and rest in order to build yourself up again. However, you may find you still have some side effects and so you may want to wait a little longer before taking a break. This will depend on when you finished your treatment and what the treatment was. It is a good idea to check with your oncologist or breast care nurse before making plans.

If you are planning to go to a hot climate, or on a winter sports holiday, do take notice of the points mentioned above about the sun.

Can I get holiday insurance if I have had breast cancer?

Yes, there is holiday and travel insurance available for people who have had cancer. If you are booking a holiday through a travel agent be sure to check the small print in any insurance cover offered to you because you may find you are excluded from some of the cover. You must always declare your breast cancer otherwise any claims could be invalidated even if you are claiming for something unrelated to breast cancer or its treatment. Sometimes holiday insurance can be more expensive after treatment for breast cancer, so you may need to shop around to get a reasonable deal. Some of the organisations listed in the Appendix will be able to provide you with more information about holiday insurance.

I have finished my treatment now. Is it safe for me to have a vaccination before I go on holiday?

Before you plan to go to any country that would require you to have any sort of vaccination or medication, you should check with the oncologist to see if it is safe to proceed. If you have recently had treatment, particularly chemotherapy, your body's defence (immune) system is quite likely to be weakened. Some vaccinations (such as for yellow fever) introduce a small amount of the virus into your body. This stimulates your body's own defence system to develop protection against the disease. If your defence system is not fully recovered from the effects of the treatment then it won't be able to react to the vaccination in the normal way, and it is likely that you will be ill. This might still apply a few months after treatment has finished.

If I need regular medication, can I take it abroad with me?

Yes, generally speaking you can, providing that you take with you a letter of explanation from your doctor. The letter should be written on headed notepaper from the hospital or practice. Make sure that you have more than enough medication in case of unforeseen delays.

Before booking a holiday, you should check with the doctor just in case the country you are going to would impose restrictions because of the type of medication you are having.

What happens if I'm taken ill while I'm away?

It is difficult to give a precise answer. It will largely depend on what the illness is and where you are. As a general guide any condition that requires hospitalisation or prolonged treatment would probably best be treated at home if you can travel. If you have doubts about any treatment offered to you while away, insist that contact is made with your doctor. If you do come back because of an illness, ensure that your family doctor and hospital doctor are informed. This is because even if the illness is not related to the cancer, there may be some treatments that are more suitable than others.

If I need to have treatment abroad, do I have to pay for it?

Yes, usually you do but there are some countries where you can receive treatment in the public health system. There are also a number of countries that have a reciprocal agreement with the UK which means that you can have treatment in that country, pay and be reimbursed by the Department of Health when you return. Check what your holiday insurance covers for healthcare abroad.

Always check before you go, perhaps with one of the organisations listed in the Appendix, and make sure you have the correct forms and know how many copies you should take with you, and so on.

SEX AND RELATIONSHIPS

Does having breast cancer mean I have to stop having a sex life?

No, it doesn't. While many people find that they are quite tired during and immediately after a course of treatment, once the side effects have passed their desire for a sexual relationship and their interest in sex returns. If you feel you want to have sex then why not? You may need to be gentle around areas that have recently been treated, for example, after breast surgery or radiotherapy to that area because you may be sore. The emotional impact of breast cancer can play a large part in when and whether or not you want to have sex, for example, women may feel low self-esteem after breast surgery or with hair loss. This is discussed later in this chapter.

Can breast cancer treatment affect my ability to have sex?

If the chemotherapy has caused your menopause to start or if you are on hormone therapies, you may experience a dry vagina as a side effect. This in itself needn't stop you having sex but it can make you a bit sore. Speak to your doctor or breast care nurse about possible ways of relieving this symptom, for example, using a lubricant.

At present I don't feel I will ever want to have sex again. Do other people feel this way?

Yes, they do. It is quite usual for people to lose their interest in sex temporarily, during and after treatment. Usually, though, their libido returns gradually.

Occasionally, the person who has had treatment wants some intimacy but their partner finds it hard to adjust and doesn't want to cuddle or touch, or in some cases, even look at the treated area. In this situation it may be helpful to take a little time to talk, maybe focus on other parts of the body and reassure your partner that they are not hurting you.

Counselling, whether individually or as a couple, may be really helpful as it can enable both parties to explore their feelings, fears and desires. This can then help them to talk to each other and work towards accepting each other's views. It might be possible to seek the help of a sex therapist to support a couple in re-discovering an intimacy that is more satisfying to both of them.

How can I ever get used to what has happened to my body?

Breast cancer always causes some physical changes to your body and you will need time to adjust to these, both physically and emotionally. Some people find that talking to their partner about how they are feeling can help. Others might prefer to see a specialist counsellor, go along to a breast cancer support group, talk to someone else who has had breast cancer and similar treatment or talk to a breast care nurse.

If you are able to share your feelings you may find it can help you to start to come to terms with what has happened, which in turn can be a big part of the recovery process.

The changes brought about by the breast cancer and/or treatment can lead to people not wanting to undress in front of anyone else, let alone have sex with another person. This is very common and for many people, adapting to the changes that have happened can take time. It is another of the reasons why many people find that talking things through can help.

I know I need to speak to someone about the way treatment has affected my body. I just can't talk to my husband about this. Who should I talk to?

Whoever you feel most comfortable with. You may want to talk to a friend or to a professional counsellor. If you have contact with a local cancer support group you might feel that is the place to go to talk through your feelings. You may choose to phone or email a breast cancer helpline or support service where you can remain anonymous.

All these self-help groups seem to be for women. Everything is pink! As a man with breast cancer, I feel a bit out of it. Who can I turn to?

Men who have breast cancer often feel marginalised because to many people breast cancer is seen as a 'woman's disease'. When men are diagnosed with breast cancer, larger cancer treatment centres will often have support systems in place to help the men to cope with both the breast cancer and this stigma. Some of the cancer support services have volunteers who are men who have had breast cancer who have been trained to offer peer support to other men. Don't be stoical! Ask for someone to talk to even if you don't really know what you want to talk about.

For many people, men and women alike, talking to someone else who has been through a similar experience is very helpful and reduces feelings of isolation and the potential for longer-term psychological problems.

There are Internet chat forums which are often international and can be helpful for people who feel isolated through their cancer. It is important to remember, however, that such forums are not often supervised and that any 'advice' given should be considered and discussed with your own medical team to see how much of it applies to you.

Some organisations, such as Breast Cancer Care, produce information specifically for men about breast cancer such as Breast Cancer Care (see Appendix).

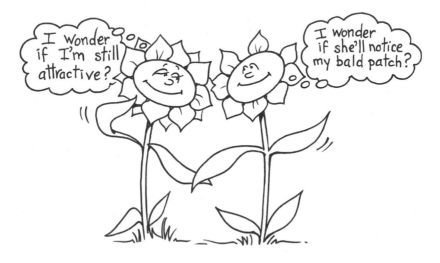

It's all too personal and I don't want to talk to anyone. Does this mean I'm not helping myself?

No. Many people feel uncomfortable talking to anyone about anything personal whether they have had cancer or not, let alone sex or relationships or about emotional matters. If you find that there are thoughts that keep going round and round in your head, then you might find it helpful to write them all down – your fears and your worries and your hopes. By transferring what is in your head onto paper, even if you tear it up and throw it away immediately afterwards, you may find it helps you to get matters clear and to free your mind to think about other things.

The current view from many research projects is that stress and future illness are greatly reduced by talking, expressing emotions, and seeking help if necessary to enable you to move on with your life.

Will I ever be able to get used to having to use a breast prosthesis?

At first, coping with the emotional effect of losing all or most of your breast through cancer can feel like a huge hurdle to get over. Using a prosthesis in your bra to provide you with the external appearance of having two intact breasts can be useful in helping you to face the outside world.

The permanent breast prostheses come in different shapes, sizes and colours. It is also possible for women who have had a partial mastectomy to get a prosthetic product.

Wearing a properly fitted prosthesis can also give you the confidence to wear evening dresses, tops with thin straps and swimwear. It is possible to buy special swimwear, for example, into which you can insert your prosthesis, knowing it will not slip out of place. The first time you try to wear something like this, you may be quite self-conscious, but it usually gets easier after the first time when you realise that people can't tell the difference between the prosthesis and the other breast.

It may take you a long time to feel that you can look at your chest and see the effects of the operation you have had. This is quite common, and is one of the reasons why talking about your feelings and fears to someone else who has been through a similar operation can be helpful.

How can I stop people from 'talking to my chest' now?

When people know you have had breast cancer surgery or any other breast cancer treatment they often, somewhat unconsciously, focus their attention on your chest when they talk to you. It is as if they are trying to decide which one is the prosthesis and which one is not, or to see if the prosthesis is a 'good one'. Annoying as it is, usually people stop doing it after a short time, but don't be afraid to point out to them what they are doing. That is often enough to stop them and after all, you don't have to put up with being stared at.

I have had reconstruction surgery but still feel like a different person. How will I ever feel able to start dating again?

Starting a new relationship after you have experienced physical changes to your body through breast cancer is not easy. Deciding when to tell and how much to say can put a great deal of pressure on you. Starting a new sexual relationship can feel almost impossible. Yet people do overcome their anxieties and fear of possible rejection and can have good, supportive relationships. As you come to terms with what has happened to you, both physically and emotionally, you are likely to find you gain in confidence which can help you to think about, and perhaps try, a new relationship.

CONTRACEPTION AND FERTILITY

I've had breast cancer treatment. Can I still take the contraceptive pill?

This will depend on a number of factors, for example, the type of breast cancer you have had and whether it was oestrogen-dependent. It may be advisable for you to use a form of contraception that doesn't involve hormones, for example, condoms. Check with your oncologist or breast care nurse.

Will taking the Pill after having breast cancer increase the chances of it returning?

There is no clear evidence to support this but your doctor may advise you against taking the Pill because of its hormone content depending on the type of breast cancer you have.

How soon after my breast cancer treatment is finished can I try to get pregnant?

That depends on the treatment you have had and should be discussed with your oncologist. Chemotherapy can cause your periods to stop for a while or permanently, which can interfere with fertility. Usually, women are advised to wait around two years after completing treatment before trying to conceive. But many hormone therapies are taken for five years and it is not advisable to get pregnant while you are on these. For some couples, it is important to balance the desire to have children with the risk of the cancer coming back.

EMPLOYMENT

Should I tell my boss and my colleagues that I've got breast cancer?

That is entirely up to you. Some people tell everyone at work what is happening, some may tell only one or two people, and others choose not to tell anyone. You will probably need to provide some explanations if you are going to need to take time off or have to keep attending hospital appointments, but legally, you do not have to tell your boss exactly what is wrong.

If you decide that you want someone at work to know about your breast cancer, but you want to be sure that the information remains confidential, remember that human resources staff and occupational health staff are bound by confidentiality and can't disclose medical details to your employer or anyone else without your permission.

Can I continue to work during my treatment?

If you feel able to continue to work then there is no reason to stop. You will need some time off to have an operation and recover and many people do take time off during chemotherapy and radiotherapy treatment. But some people do continue to work.

A lot will depend on your work schedule: some employers are quite flexible and if you are self-employed you may find it easier to 'work around' appointments. It also depends on how emotionally and physically draining your job is. Some people are able to work shorter hours or to take an occasional day or two off (for example, around the time you have chemotherapy) rather than stopping work altogether. If you are continuing on hormone therapy for some time, you may feel able to go back to work full-time.

Sometimes the pressure of needing to earn an income is difficult to balance against allowing yourself to recover from what can be pretty tough treatments. Only you can decide what is right for you.

Could I lose my job if I need to take time off work because of my cancer or treatment?

Anyone who has cancer is protected by the Disability Discrimination Act. This means that you can't be sacked just because you have cancer. Providing you tell them about what is happening, employers are expected in law to make all reasonable efforts to help you to continue to work, if you wish to. They should also not discriminate against you, for example, if you apply for promotion. If you have any concerns about your employment rights, you should talk to a union representative, the human resources department or occupational health staff, and for more information about the law contact your local Citizens Advice Bureau or Macmillan Cancer Support. Breast Cancer Care has recently published an Employment Charter (see Appendix for all contact information).

I'm unemployed. When I go for a new job do I have to say that I have had breast cancer?

If you are asked about your health you should answer truthfully. Although all employers are bound by the Disability Discrimination Act, you could present the truth in such a way as to try to allay some of the concerns an employer may have. For example, you could say that you have had treatment for breast cancer, that you have regular check-ups and that currently you are cancer free.

If you don't say anything and the truth comes out later on, you run the risk of being dismissed no matter how long you have worked in the job, or how well you carry out your work.

FINANCE

Am I entitled to sick pay if I can't work for a few months?

Each employer will have their own sick pay arrangements. Some only pay the legal minimum, while others are more generous. If you have been paying National Insurance contributions then you are likely to be able to receive Statutory Sick Pay (SSP). This is payable for a total of 28 weeks. If you are off sick for longer than 28 weeks, your local Benefits Agency will usually transfer you to a longer-term benefit which is called Invalidity Benefit.

How can I find out if I am entitled to any welfare benefits?

It is not easy to answer this question as benefits and allowances change regularly. For specific and detailed financial advice, you should speak to your personnel or welfare officer at work if there is one, or to the hospital social worker, or to your local Citizens Advice Bureau or Benefits Agency (Department of Work and Pensions).

Macmillan Cancer Support has a specific information line which can provide up-to-date information about benefits and other financial matters (see Appendix for contact details).

My son may have to give up work or take a long time off to look after me. Can he claim benefits?

You should seek specialist advice to find out if your son is entitled to any welfare benefits if he stops work. Individual employers may be willing to discuss ways in which carers can take extended leave without losing their salary, or they may keep their job open for them for a period of time.

If your son has not paid enough National Insurance contributions to ensure a full pension, he can protect his state pension if he is off work caring for you. In this case he could apply for Home Responsibilities Protection. Contact one of the organisations mentioned earlier in this section or Carers UK (see Appendix) for more details.

Can I get life insurance if I have had breast cancer?

Different companies have different rules about this. Some companies will sell you life insurance if you have been disease free for a certain period of time, or if your cancer was an early stage cancer. Other companies will only insure you for an extremely high premium, or will not consider insuring you at all, regardless of the type and stage of cancer.

You are unlikely to be able to get life insurance if it has been less than two years since you had cancer. Between two and seven years after having cancer some companies will insure you, but will probably charge a higher premium. If you are seven years cancer-and-recurrence-free, you will probably find you can get life insurance without incurring penalties.

Both Cancerbackup and Macmillan Cancer Support have information about this and other financial matters.

I'm the main wage earner. I haven't been able to work full time for some months and I'm worried we won't be able to pay the mortgage and all the bills. Where can I turn to for help and advice?

Talk to your bank or building society; they should be able to advise you about your mortgage. Many of the utility companies have schemes to help people spread out their bill payments so it's worth talking to them about this. You may also be able to claim some welfare benefits, even in the short term, so contact one of the agencies referred to in the previous questions. Don't feel bad about this – you have been paying into national schemes for many years!

Will the fact that I have had breast cancer affect my chances of getting a mortgage?

You are just as likely to be able to get a mortgage as anyone else even if it has been less than two years since you had cancer, but it may not have any life insurance cover (see previous question). The type and terms of the mortgage can sometimes depend on whether you are the sole person taking out the mortgage or if it is a joint one.

Can I get private medical cover if I have had breast cancer?

Like all insurance, most private medical insurance will have certain exclusions, so that in some situations you will not be able to claim. It is possible that if you have had breast cancer you will get medical insurance but it may state that it will not pay out for anything to do with the cancer in the future. It is also possible that your premium will be increased once you have had breast cancer.

7 | The future

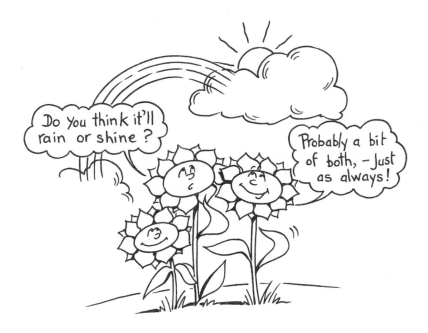

Questions about the longer-term effects of breast cancer can be very difficult for someone to ask. Many of them are concerned with subjects which are rarely discussed – the possible recurrence of disease after treatment and living with incurable illness. This chapter discusses these questions, but also looks at the strengths that some people find as a result of having had breast cancer.

What are the chances of my breast cancer coming back?

The majority of people treated for breast cancer will never have any problems in the future. Some types of breast cancer are known to have a greater tendency to reappear later, either back in the breast or chest area or elsewhere in the body; other types are less likely to do this.

Even if the type of breast cancer you have had is one that is likely to recur, no one can tell you for certain when and how this might happen. And there will always be people who don't get a recurrence of their breast cancer, even though statistically this was thought to be likely.

What do I do if cancer comes back?

When cancer comes back it can be devastating after all the treatment you have had before, and also the fact that you may have enjoyed a long time with no problems. A recurrence will mean different things depending on where in the body it has come back. Breast cancer that has come back or spread can still be treated, and some people are able to live with advanced breast cancer for several years.

Support is available from all the sources mentioned in Chapter 6.

I sometimes feel that there is no point planning for the future. Do other people who have breast cancer get like this?

Yes, this is a common feeling. In facing up to breast cancer many people find they have strengths they might never have known about, and discover things about themselves that they might never otherwise have had the chance to do. Having breast cancer can lead to people taking stock of their lives and making changes that they might never have dared to do.

That is not to underestimate the effects of breast cancer. For many people it is the worst and most devastating experience of their lives. Being forced to confront breast cancer is likely to cause some emotional distress, some psychological stress and could have physical implications that could never have been imagined. Yet often, as time goes on, the initial shock waves subside and the side effects of treatment pass, and people are able to think once more about things in their lives other than their breast cancer.

The cancer has caused lots of change in my life, most of which I
would not have planned. I actually now feel like making major
changes of my own free will! Is this a common thing?

For some people, the enforced break in their regular routine that comes through having breast cancer and treatment is like being given a chance to review things. It can help you to realise that change is long overdue. Having had the courage to face your illness you may find that other changes are much less daunting. Perhaps you finally decide to make changes in an unsuccessful relationship or unrewarding job, or in the balance of work and home life. Of course the cancer may make you realise that you like your life just as it is.

Whatever the outcome of taking stock, many people come to view their breast cancer journey as a 'wake up call' that leads them to want to make the most of the future.

I really can't stop thinking that my breast cancer will come
back. Does this worry ever go away?

The fear of having a recurrence of their breast cancer is one that most people have. Often, the longer it is since you had the original cancer, the more the fear reduces, although it is unlikely ever to go away completely.

Some people say that the first thing they imagine whenever they have an ache or pain is that it is the breast cancer returning, even if deep down they know that this is unlikely. The other key time when people say they worry that their breast cancer might have recurred is when they are coming up to the time of a check-up with the surgeon or oncologist. Even if you are feeling fine, it is quite common to have anxieties about the check-up and wonder if something new will be found. Some people don't realise their raised anxiety level is connected to the appointment date, but if you notice your own stress levels rising without an obvious reason, you may find this is the link.

What all this means is that on some level, conscious or not, most people do fear recurrence from time to time. Sometimes a short course of counselling can be helpful to address this, reduce stress and develop some management strategies.

I think about the cancer coming back all the time. It even keeps me awake at night. What can I do to help myself?

One thing you can do is to share your thoughts with someone else. If you keep them bottled up inside, the worry can build up and get quite out of proportion. You might find that someone who has had breast cancer would be a good person to talk to as it is likely they will have had similar feelings from time to time. This could be someone from a breast cancer support group or a professional counsellor. A few sessions can make a big difference by helping you to find practical strategies to manage your worries.

If you are worried that a new cancer might be developing you can arrange to see the oncologist or surgeon, by bringing your regular check-up appointment forward if necessary.

Because I've had breast cancer, does this mean that I could get another type of cancer in the future?

No, this is not likely. The only exception is in women whose breast cancer is caused by an inherited faulty gene. They might have a higher risk of ovarian cancer but this will only affect very few people overall. Generally, you should have been told about this when you were first diagnosed.

I am determined to do all I can to stop the cancer coming back. What can I do to prevent getting a recurrence?

There is little anyone can do to guarantee that they do not get any recurrence. Your best plan is to improve your general health, by following the suggestions outlined in previous chapters about eating a balanced diet, limiting alcohol and taking regular exercise. Not only may this help reduce the chances of a recurrence, but your good health can also help you enjoy life to the full.

I have asked everyone on the team for their opinion about my future. No one seems able to give me a definite answer. Why can no one be certain about my future?

One thing that everyone who has had breast cancer wants to hear is that their cancer is cured and that it won't come back. While this will actually be the case for the majority of people, it isn't possible to predict this for each individual. Cancer does not always follow the 'rules' – so no one is really able to provide a cast-iron guarantee that their breast cancer won't ever return.

When you ask about breast cancer being cured, why do people talk about five-year and ten-year survival figures?

Researchers quote survival statistics, usually referring to people being free of cancer five or ten years after it was diagnosed. These are only really of value for statistical purposes and to show possible trends in the population as a whole.

People who have breast cancer will often ask 'what are my chances?' but care should be taken when interpreting statistics. If you are told that you have a 90% chance of being cancer-free in five years, time, what does this mean for you as an individual? Do you focus on this and ignore the other 10% chance? Or, if you are told you have a 40% chance of being alive and well in five years' time, will you feel sure you will be amongst the 40% and not the other 60%? Remember, statistics relate to whole populations, not to individuals.

What is known is that because breast cancer is so common in the 'developed world' there has been plenty of research, and there are now many different treatments which have much greater success in treating the disease. If, for example, you look at the statistics for a particular type of breast cancer 20 years ago, which then had a poor prognosis (outlook), the same type of breast cancer today is likely to be more effectively treated. So if you are looking at statistics, you need the most recent figures and to compare similar types of breast cancer and treatment regimens. Ask your breast care nurse, specialist or a breast cancer charity where to find this information.

I've got plenty of good information from the Internet. There's a lot there about 'survivorship': what does this mean?

Survivorship is a term that refers to quality of life after a cancer diagnosis. When it comes to breast cancer, there are many, many personal stories about being a survivor, about fighting cancer and about getting on with life. You will find them in articles, photographs, chatroom forums and hospital or community-led support initiatives. You may or may not find it helpful to read some of these and perhaps to share in the forums.

Increasingly, as more and more people live and are well after breast cancer, there are conferences specifically for survivors held in different countries. It's like being part of an exclusive club and for many people these conferences are affirming and confidence-boosting experiences. Some of the organisations listed in the Appendix will be able to tell you about these events.

There are times when I feel fine and then there are times when I am scared that I might die from my breast cancer. Is this common?

Yes, it is very common. Even several years after having breast cancer you may feel like this. It is something that relatives, friends and health professionals tend not to realise, particularly if it is some time since your treatment has finished, and this can make it hard to talk about your worries. Many people will have put your breast cancer experience to the back of their minds and may be surprised to hear you mention it, unless perhaps you are just about to go for a check-up.

It is really important that you do find someone to talk to about your feelings. You are not alone and there are many people who could identify with you and with your experience, but these may not be relatives or close friends. The Appendix lists organisations that can help you to find support.

LIVING WITH RECURRENCE

Breast cancer may return in the area around the breast or in other organs of the body. If the breast cancer comes back in the breast or the skin of the chest it is called a **local recurrence**. If it spreads nearby, for example, to lymph nodes draining the breast area such as the axilla (armpit), it is called a **regional recurrence**.

Metastases are cancer cells that have spread from the original, or primary, cancer. If the breast cancer has spread to another part of the body this is called **distant metastasis** or secondary breast cancer.

Tests can show that metastases are from the spread of breast cancer rather than being a new, different cancer. When breast cancer has spread from the breast to another part of the body, the cells in the new area are breast cancer cells. For example, under a microscope, cells from a breast cancer that have spread to the lungs will look like breast cancer cells and they will behave like breast cancer, whereas the cells making up a primary lung cancer will look like and behave like lung cancer cells.

Does it make any difference to the treatment if I have a recurrence of the original breast cancer or a new primary cancer?

Yes, the treatment may be quite different for a primary cancer than for a secondary breast cancer. That is one of the reasons why it is very important to have tests done to find out which it is before embarking on a long course of treatment.

If my breast cancer does come back, can it be treated successfully?

If the breast cancer comes back in the breast or chest wall area it can still be cured. But once breast cancer has spread away from these areas to other parts of the body it can no longer be cured, although it can still be treated with the view to halting its growth for as long as possible – and this could be years.

Are the same options available for treating secondary breast cancer as there are for treating primary cancer?

The treatments may be similar. For example, secondary breast cancer may be treated with chemotherapy, hormone therapy or radiotherapy and occasionally surgery. This will depend on several factors including:

- the type of primary breast cancer;
- how the primary breast cancer was treated (particularly what radiotherapy, chemotherapy and hormone therapy drugs you have had before);
- how long ago you had your initial treatment;
- where the secondary breast cancer is in your body (it may be in more than one area).

Is there a limit to how much treatment I can have?

There are limits to how often some forms of treatment can be used. For example, if you have had a high dose of radiotherapy to your breast/chest, there will be a point at which you could not have any more radiotherapy in that area without causing permanent damage to the tissues. However, you could have radiotherapy to another part of your body. With chemotherapy you can usually have more, but you will not have too much of one drug very soon after you had it previously, and you may need to have different drugs than before because of the side effects.

My wife has secondary breast cancer and the doctor recently talked to us about palliative treatment. What does he mean by this?

Palliative treatment or **palliative care** is a term that describes the use of treatment to control or alleviate symptoms, such as pain, rather than aiming to reduce or get rid of the cancer completely.

Some people live for a number of years having regular palliative treatment to keep cancer symptoms at bay. Not being able to be cured does not mean that you (or the health professionals) give up. There are many things that can be done to help your wife to continue to live normally.

What will happen to me if there are no more treatment options?

Breast cancer is one of the most well-researched and documented types of cancer. This means that whatever kind of breast cancer you have, there is likely to be information available to doctors to help look for treatment options.

There are many different clinical trials taking place at any time and a significant number of these will be related to breast cancer. If there are no more regular treatment options available, there might still be a trial taking place for which you are eligible.

If you are not eligible for any trials then palliative care may still be effective at controlling symptoms for some time.

I can't believe that my breast cancer can't be cured. Isn't there something I can try that might still cure it?

It is very difficult to be told you have secondary breast cancer which cannot be cured. It is quite normal to feel that there must be something new you could try which gives you renewed hope.

Remember some people live with secondary breast cancer for many years and new treatments are developed all the time. If you do decide you want to try something else, here are a few things you could do.

- Get a second opinion from another specialist to see if they have any suggestions.

- Find out if there is a clinical trial of a treatment for the type of breast cancer you have (see Chapter 3).

- Certain complementary therapies might help you to feel as though you are continuing to do something active in terms of helping yourself. Several are described in Chapter 4. However, beware of 'miracle cures' as there is no evidence that they will be able to cure, or control, breast cancer.

How long have I got left to live?

This is what most people want to know when they have secondary breast cancer. It is also almost impossible to answer and will depend on where the secondary breast cancer is and how it is responding to treatment. Breast cancer can be unpredictable so it is very difficult for doctors to be precise but they can give you an approximate idea if you want them to. Even then you may exceed their expectations, so beware of putting too much store by what is really only an educated guess.

Throughout this book we have tried to provide realistic answers to some of the myriad of questions that we, as cancer professionals, have been asked to answer over many years in this field. We know that research is on-going, that cancer treatments continue to be developed and that options for palliative care are also improving all the time. Our hope is to have provided you with accurate information to guide you and support you both now and in the future. Always remember that nearly three-quarters of people are still alive and well ten years after a diagnosis of breast cancer.

| Glossary

Terms in *italics* also appear in the glossary.

adjuvant (additional) therapies cancer treatments besides surgery. Main adjuvant therapies are *chemotherapy*, *radiotherapy* and *hormone therapy*.

allopathy a system of treatment where a condition is treated with its opposite, unlike homeopathy. Orthodox medicine is allopathic.

anaemia shortage of red blood cells, leading to a lack of oxygen in the tissues.

analgesia painkilling drugs.

anti-emetic a drug to relieve nausea, or feeling sick.

axilla the armpit.

axillary dissection surgery to remove lymph nodes in the armpit region.

benign describes a *tumour* which is not *malignant* and will not spread to other tissues.

biopsy a sample of living tissue taken for examination.

blood count the number of a blood component (e.g. *white blood cells*) in a sample of blood.

BRCA1 an inherited faulty gene which can mean an increased risk of developing breast, ovarian or bowel cancer.

BRCA2 an inherited faulty gene which can mean an increased risk of developing breast, ovarian, prostate, male breast cancer and malignant melanoma.

breast aware being conscious of what is normal for oneself, so that even small changes in a breast are noticeable.

breast conserving surgery cancer surgery where the major part of a breast is left intact (e.g. lumpectomy, *wide local excision*).

carcinoma a *malignant* growth.

catheter a tube inserted in the body to supply or remove liquid.

central venous catheter (a Hickman line) a tube supplying liquid into a vein in the upper body.

chemotherapy drug treatment to destroy cancer cells.

chromosome the part of each cell that contains DNA.

clinical oncologist a doctor who deals specifically with treating patients with cancer with radiotherapy (*radiotherapist*).

clinical trial a test for a new drug or treatment, whereby the outcome in a group of patients who take the drug is compared with those of a similar group who do not take it.

complementary therapy a healing treatment usually from a tradition outside Western medicine which can be used alongside orthodox treatment.

core biopsy a small section of tissue taken for analysis.

CT scan (Computed Tomography) an X-ray method that uses three-dimensional images analysed by a computer to show structures within the body.

cyst a small, usually hard, fluid-filled *benign* growth in the tissues.

cytotoxic poisonous to cells.

detoxification a process whereby potentially harmful waste products are removed from the body.

differentiation the process whereby cells become part of recognisable tissues, e.g. bone cells or liver cells.

distant metastasis a cancer which has spread to a part of the body away from the primary site.

ductal carcinoma in situ a pre-invasive cancer in the cells of the breast ducts (see Figure 1).

endocrine gland any gland which secretes hormones into the bloodstream, e.g. the ovaries, pituitary, pancreas.

endocrine therapy treatment using hormones as drugs.

familial describes conditions which 'run in families' and which we may be prone to because of genetics.

fibroadenoma a benign *tumour* of glandular and fibrous tissue. Most breast lumps in young women are fibroadenomas.

fibrosis thickening and scarring of tissue caused by injury or inflammation.

fine needle aspiration cytology the removal of cells for examination by suction, using a needle and syringe.

first-degree relative someone related directly to you by blood: a parent, sibling or child.

gene a unit of heredity, coded on the DNA in the nucleus of cells, which we inherit from our parents and pass to our children.

grade in breast cancer, the degree of cellular change in a cancer from normal breast tissue. Breast cancer can be grade 1, 2 or 3, with grade 1 showing least change.

granulocyte-colony stimulating factor a circulating hormonal substance that controls the growth of some of the white cells of the blood.

HER-2 positive breast cancer one which responds to a protein called HER-2 (human epidermal growth factor receptor 2), and which is treated by drugs which target the protein.

hereditary describes a feature or condition which is passed from parent to child.

Hickman line see *central venous catheter.*

holistic describes an approach to treatment which takes into account more than just the physical body.

hormone chemical messengers that play a part in regulating growth and reproduction.

hormone therapy drug treatment using hormones.

incidence the number of cases occurring in a given population during a set period, usually expressed as cases per 1000 or 10 000 per year.

intravenous infusion passing a liquid into a vein, where it is rapidly dispersed around the body.

invasive ductal carcinoma a cancer in the breast duct which has the ability to spread.

invasive lobular carcinoma a cancer in the lobes of the breast with the ability to spread.

immune system the body's natural defences against infection.

implant a manufactured, usually silicone, device which is put surgically into the breast to enlarge it or to replace tissue that has been removed.

implanted port a *catheter* system with a catheter inserted into a large vein above the heart with a port under the skin into which fluids can be injected.

isotope bone scan the use of radioactive isotopes which can be safely introduced into the body and which tend to concentrate in the bone, and can be measured with a gamma camera.

local recurrence the re-growth of a cancer in the primary site after treatment.

lumpectomy an operation to remove a breast lump with a small amount of surrounding healthy tissue.

lymph a watery liquid which drains from tissues into *lymph nodes* and then into the bloodstream.

lymph nodes small oval bodies, up to 2 cm in length, situated in groups along the lymph draining vessels. They are packed with lymphocytes, and produce antibodies to fight infection.

lymph node negative signifies that breast cancer has not spread to local *lymph nodes*.

lymph node positive a breast cancer that has spread to local *lymph nodes*.

lymphatic system the system of lymphatic drainage vessels and *lymph nodes* which are found in the groin, armpit, neck, abdomen and chest.

lymphoedema swelling of the tissues caused by poor lymphatic drainage.

malignant describes a *tumour* that is cancerous.

mammogram literally 'a picture of the breast' – a 'soft' X-ray of the breast used to detect dense areas of tissue which may be *tumours*.

manual lymph drainage massage specifically to aid the body disperse *lymphoedema*.

mastectomy surgical removal of the breast.

medical oncologist a doctor who specialises in treating cancer with drugs or hormones.

metastasis the spread or transfer of cancer from the original site to another place in the body where the disease process starts up. It usually occurs through the bloodstream or *lymphatic system*. Cancers at a new site are **metastases**.

metastatic breast cancer cancer that has spread from the breast to sites elsewhere in the body, such as the bone or liver.

MRI scan (magnetic resonance imaging) a method of body scanning which shows details of soft tissues that other scanning methods do not.

multi-disciplinary team (MDT) the group of medical staff working on a case: in breast cancer, this will include the surgeon, *oncologist*, *radiologist*, *pathologist*, breast care nurse and others.

neo-adjuvant therapy the use of drug therapies (*chemotherapy* or *hormone therapy*) before surgery.

oesophagus the muscular tube which takes food from the throat to the stomach, passing through the diaphragm.

oestrogen a steroid sex hormone secreted mainly by the ovaries, also used in HRT to treat menopausal symptoms.

oestrogen receptor positive breast cancer (oestrogen positive breast cancer) a breast cancer which grows in response to *oestrogen.*

omega-3 one of three essential fatty acids, required by the body, which are taken from food.

oncologist a cancer specialist.

palliative treatment (palliative care) treatment that relieves symptoms but does not cure their cause.

paraben chemical added to cosmetic products and food packaging as a preservative.

pathologists those studying the causes of disease.

peripherally inserted central catheter (PICC) a tube inserted into a vein in the arm, to supply liquid or take blood.

physiotherapist a healthcare professional who uses physical methods to restore function to a disabled part of the body with, for example, active or passive exercise, heat treatment, massage or *ultrasound.*

phyto-oestrogen a hormone-like substance found in plants which mimics the effects of human *oestrogen.*

platelet a blood component which forms clots.

primary breast cancer cancer which originates in the breast.

progesterone hormone secreted by the ovary and the placenta, involved in the menstrual cycle and pregnancy, and used in HRT. Synthetic progesterone is called progestogen.

progesterone receptor positive breast cancer (progesterone positive breast cancer) a breast cancer which grows in response to oestrogen.

prognosis the likely outcome of a disease, the life expectancy.

prosthesis a false body part; in breast cancer, a manufactured breast form designed to fit into a bra to replace either the whole breast or part of it.

radiologist a doctor specialising in medical imaging, skilled in interpreting, for example, X-ray, CT scan, MRI, PET scan films.

radiotherapist a doctor who treats cancer by ionising radiation (also called a *clinical oncologist*).

reconstruction the rebuilding of the breast after mastectomy as realistically as possible.

red blood cells component of the blood which make it red, and which carry oxygen from the lungs to the tissues.

regional recurrence a cancer which comes back in the same region of the body after treatment.

risk factors features which, in the population as a whole, are seen to affect the chances of having a disease; for example, being female is a risk factor for having breast cancer.

screening the routine examination of numbers of apparently healthy people to identify those with a particular disease at an early stage.

secondaries (secondary breast cancer, metastases) cancers occurring at a site remote from the original, primary site, from which it has spread.

secondary breast cancer in the bone a breast cancer which has spread to the bone.

sentinel lymph node biopsy a method of checking the *sentinel nodes* for possible cancer spread to the *lymph nodes*, which is an accurate way of predicting general spread to lymph nodes.

sentinel node the *lymph node* presumed to be the first to which a cancer will spread.

seroma a collection of serum that builds up in the spaces left behind after surgery. Serum is the colourless liquid in blood.

simulator a machine that simulates a process, as in *radiotherapy* treatment.

stage the degree to which a cancer has progressed. Staging is important in indicating the best treatment and likely outcome.

systemic involving the whole of a body system, for example, the circulation, the digestive system, the nervous system. The opposite of systemic is **local**.

targeted therapy drug treatment aimed at the agents other than hormones which make cancers grow.

TP53 An inherited gene mutation, or faulty gene, which can bring an increased risk of developing breast cancer and a very rare syndrome that increases the risk of other cancers, including brain tumours and malignant melanoma.

Traditional Chinese Medicine (TCM) comprises acupuncture, Chinese herbs and Tui Na, a physical therapy.

ultrasound scan a method of body imaging based on sound reflection. It is very safe and is used in pregnancy.

white blood cells component of the blood, part of the *immune system*, of which there are several types, all involved in fighting infection.

wide local excision breast cancer surgery where up to a quarter of the breast is removed. It takes more away than does a *lumpectomy*, but less than *mastectomy*.

Appendix:
Sources of further help and information

BOOKS

There are now many books available about cancer and its treatment, and more on complementary therapies or ways of reducing stress and increasing well-being. A browse through the health section of a large bookshop or your local library will help you to select a book which suits you. Always check when a book was published to make sure the information is up-to-date and also the qualifications of the authors so you know that the content is from a reputable source.

WEBSITES

If you venture onto the world-wide web you need to be selective: using key words such as 'breast cancer' or 'breast cancer treatment' will produce thousands of sites. Some of these are extremely good but others list ineffective or harmful therapies, often expensive or not available in the UK. Good starting points in the UK are Breast Cancer Care or Cancerbackup and other general or specific cancer organisations listed here. Another might be the American Cancer Society on www.cancer.org, although treatments and opinions on how some cancers should be treated vary on different sides of the Atlantic. Again, you should look at the source of the information and when it was last updated.

If you find something on the web that you think may help you, print it off and discuss it with your doctor or one of the staff caring for you. They will be able to give you advice about whether it is available, appropriate for you and effective.

ORGANISATIONS

The organisations listed here represent a range of national information sources and support networks for people affected by breast cancer. Local libraries and telephone directories may provide further information about regional or local sources of support. We include a list of national professional bodies who set standards for complementary therapists and who can provide information about qualified therapists in your area.

The information listed is that provided by each organisation to the authors and is correct at the time of going to print.

Cancer care and support

Breakthrough Breast Cancer
Weston House
246 High Holborn
London WC1V 7EX
Freephone: 0808 0100 200
Email: info@breakthrough.org.uk
Website: www.breakthrough.org.uk
Breakthrough Breast Cancer is the leading charity committed to fighting breast cancer through research, campaigning and education. Our work – funding scientific research; campaigning for improvements in access to diagnosis, treatment and care; and promoting breast awareness and breast screening to encourage early diagnosis – aims to fulfil our vision of a future free from the fear of breast cancer for everyone. For more information on breast cancer or a free copy of our booklets on breast cancer risk factors, having a family history of breast cancer or Breakthrough's Best Treatment Guidelines phone us or visit our website.

Breast Cancer Campaign
Clifton Centre
110 Clifton Street
London EC2A 4HT
Tel: 020 7749 3700
Email: info@breastcancercampaign.org
Website: www.breastcancercampaign.org
Breast Cancer Campaign is the only charity that specialises in funding independent breast cancer research throughout the UK. It aims to fund research which looks at improving diagnosis and treatment, better understanding how breast cancer develops and ultimately either curing the disease or preventing it.

Breast Cancer Care
5–13 Great Suffolk Street
London SE1 0NS
Freephone: 0808 800 6000
Textphone: 0808 800 6001
Tel: 020 7384 2984
Website: www.breastcancercare.org.uk

Breast Cancer Care is the UK's leading provider of information, practical assistance and emotional support for anyone affected by breast cancer. Every year it gives support to over 20,000 people with breast cancer or breast health concerns through their helpline, peer support and other direct services. In addition it is contacted almost two million times a year through its publications, website and outreach work. All services are free.

Breast Cancer Care is committed to campaigning for better treatment and support for people with breast cancer and their families.

For information, emotional support and details of services, call the free helpline.

Breast Cancer Care's website has an email enquiries service called 'Ask the nurse', along with forums and live chat sessions where you can share your views with people in a similar situation. For more information about these services and other online support visit the website.

In addition, BCC centres provide one-to-one support and other services, including Healthy Living days, Living with Secondary Breast Cancer courses, HeadStrong for people experiencing hair loss from chemotherapy, and Younger Women's Forums for the under-45s.

Contact details for the centres:

North and Midlands
Tel: 0845 077 1893
Email: nrc@breastcancercare.org.uk

London and South
Tel: 0845 077 1895
Email: src@breastcancercare.org.uk

Scotland
Tel: 0845 077 1892
Email: sco@breastcancercare.org.uk

Cymru/Wales
Tel: 0845 077 1894
Email: cym@breastcancercare.org.uk

Breast Cancer Care also has a wide range of publications to guide you through from diagnosis to living well after treatment. You can download or order these from the website or call the helpline for booklets, factsheets or a printed order form.

Breast Cancer Haven
Effie Road
London
SW6 1TB
Tel: 020 7384 0000
Email: info@breastcancerhaven.org.uk
Website: www.breastcancerhaven.org.uk
*Being diagnosed with breast cancer
and undergoing treatment affects a
person both physically and
emotionally. Breast Cancer Haven
offers a free programme of care to help
patients and those supporting them
during this difficult time. Havens are
welcoming places staffed by a specialist
team that provides support,
information and complementary
therapies before, during and after
medical treatment. Breast Cancer
Haven believes no one should have to
face breast cancer alone and is
committed to opening a network of
Havens across the UK.*

Cancer Black Care
79 Acton Lane
London NW10 8UT
Tel: 020 8961 4151
Fax: 020 8961 4152
Email: info@cancerblackcare.org
Website: www.cancerblackcare.org
*Cancer Black Care provides a
comprehensive support service to **all**
members of the community who are
affected by cancer. It offers a safe,
confidential, neutral place, where
service users, carers, families and
friends can meet to support each
other's cultural and emotional needs.
As every family is unique, the service
is committed to the interest of our
service users and their family,
remaining sensitive to cultural and
ethnic diversity.*

*Cancer Black Care aims to enhance
the quality of life by reducing fears,
tension, bitterness and misunder-
standing. It assists and encourages
individuals to discuss and reach
important decisions which affect them
and their families. It provides support
throughout and beyond the illness.
Anyone in the community affected by
cancer has the opportunity of
benefiting from the wide range of
services including counselling,
information, family support, welfare
benefit advice, financial support and
monthly user-led support group
meetings.*

Cancerbackup
3 Bath Place
Rivington Street
London EC2A 3JR
Freephone: 0808 800 1234
(Mon–Fri 9 am–8 pm)
Admin: 020 7696 9003
Website: www.cancerbackup.org.uk
*Cancerbackup is the only UK charity
that specialises in high-quality
information on all types of cancer.
Its mission is to give cancer patients
and their families the information,
understanding and support they need
to reduce the fear and uncertainty of*

cancer. Able to answer any question on any cancer, the charity offers independent information, practical advice and support to people affected by cancer via a freephone helpline staffed by specialist cancer nurses. There is also a comprehensive range of booklets, leaflets and factsheets, an award-winning website, and a network of local cancer information centres staffed by specialist cancer nurses.

Telephone support and written information is available in several languages. It also has a website for teenagers with cancer: www.click4tic.org.uk *and a website where people affected by cancer can share their experiences:* www.whatnow.org.uk

Cancerbackup Scotland
Suite 2
3rd Floor
Argyle Street
Glasgow G2 8BH
Tel: 0141 223 7676

Cancerbackup Jersey
The Lido Medical Centre
St Saviour's Road
St Saviour, Jersey JE2 7LA
Freephone: 0800 735 0275
Tel: 01534 498 189

Cancer Counselling Trust
2 Wakley Street
London EC1V 7LT
Tel: 020 7704 1137
Email: support@cctrust.org.uk
Website: www.cancercounselling.org.uk
The Cancer Counselling Trust is the only national charity with the remit to provide free specialist counselling for those affected by cancer and their family and friends.

Formed in 1999, the charity has grown organically from a small base, attaining a reputation for excellence.

Their counsellors are all fully qualified and have worked in the field of cancer for decades and are specialists in their work. This specialism allows clients to feel understood and supported not only in what they're going through but in understanding stages of diagnosis, different types of treatment and the impact varying types of cancer can have.

Cancer Equality
27–29 Vauxhall Grove
London, SW8 1SY
Tel: 020 7735 7888
Fax: 020 7820 1115
Email: info@cancerequality.org.uk
Website: www.cancerequality.org.uk
*Cancer Equality works to improve
access to cancer information and
support services for Black and
Minority Ethnic (BME) and Refugee
communities and address the gaps in
provision of culturally appropriate
information and services. It produces*
The Directory of Cancer
Information available in Ethnic
Minority Languages, *and culturally
appropriate dietary information for
cancer patients from BME
communities.*

*Cancer Equality raises awareness
about all aspects of cancer within the
BME and Refugee communities and
acts as a central resource of cancer
information and good practice for the
target group. It also works in
partnership with communities, health
professionals and users to influence
service providers to meet their needs.*

*'Cancer Equality Works for
Excellence in Cancer Care.'*

Cancer Research UK
61 Lincoln's Inn Fields
London
WC2A 3PX
Tel: 020 7242 0200
Email: supporter.services@cancer.org.uk
Website: www.cancerresearchuk.org
*Cancer Research UK is the world's
leading independent organisation
dedicated to cancer research. It
supports research into all aspects of
cancer through the work of more than
4250 scientists, doctors and nurses.*

Carers UK
Ruth Pitter House
20–25 Glasshouse Yard
London EC1A 4JT
Carersline:
Freephone: 0808 808 7777
(Wed–Thu, 10 am–12 noon, 2–4 pm)
Email: info@carersuk.org
Website: www.carersuk.org.uk
*Carers UK offers confidential advice
and information to any carer by phone
or letter from experts on welfare
rights, benefits and community care
issues. There is a UK-wide network
of offices, branches and individuals
offering support to carers.*

Chai Cancer Care

144–146 Great North Way
London
NW4 1EH
Tel: 020 8202 2211
Freephone: 0808 808 4567
Fax: 020 8202 2111
Email: info@chaicancercare.org
*Chai Cancer Care is the Jewish
Community's cancer support
organisation providing an extensive
range of services to cancer patients
and their families which include
counselling, support groups and
complementary therapies. In addition
there are a range of physical activities,
yoga, pilates and gentle exercise
groups. There are social activities
each week. A range of expert advice
and educational programmes are also
available.*

Counsel and Care

Twyman House
16 Bonny Street
London
NW1 9PG
Advice Line: 0845 300 7585 (calls at
local rate) (Mon–Fri, 10 am–4 pm,
except Wed, 10 am–1 pm)
Email: advice@counselandcare.org.uk
Website: www.counselandcare.org.uk
*Counsel and Care is a national charity
aimed at getting the best care and
support for older people, their families,
carers and involved professionals.
There is a national advice service, and
the charity provides 43 factsheets*

*which are available to download free of
charge from the website. The charity
can make small one-off grants for
essential items.*

Crossroads Caring for Carers

Crossroads Association
10 Regent Place
Rugby
Warwickshire CV21 2PN
Tel: 0845 450 0350
Fax: 0845 450 6556
Website: www.crossroads.org.uk
*Crossroads operates 150 local schemes
in the UK which provide practical
support for carers where and when it is
most needed – usually in the home. A
trained Carer Support Worker will take
over from the carer to give them 'time
to be themselves'. Over 4.6 million
care hours are provided every year to
more than 35,000 carers. You can find
your local scheme from the Crossroads
website.*

Disabled Living Foundation

380–384 Harrow Road
London W9 2HU
Tel: 020 7289 6111
Helpline: 0870 603 9177
(Mon–Fri, 10 am–4 pm)
Fax: 020 7266 2922
Email: info@dlf.org.uk
Website: www.dlf.org.uk
*National resource for information
about equipment to help people with
a disability to carry out daily living
activities.*

GaysCan
Tel: 020 8368 9027
(Mon–Sat, 10 am–8 pm)
Website: gayscan@blotholm.org.uk
National helpline offering confidential help and support to gay men living with cancer, their partners, families and friends.

Hospice Information
Help the Hospices
Hospice House
34–44 Britannia Street
London WC1X 9JG

St Christopher's Hospice
51–59 Lawrie Park Road
London SE26 6DZ
Tel: 0807 903 3903
(calls charged at national rates)
Fax: 020 7278 1021
Email: info@hospiceinformation.info
Website: www.hospiceinformation.info
Hospice Information is provided by Help the Hospices and St Christopher's Hospice.
    It is an information service about UK and international hospices and palliative care. It publishes a directory of hospice and palliative care services which provides details of hospices, home care teams, and hospital support teams in the UK and the Republic of Ireland.
    For details of local services, including hospice services for children, write, email or telephone. Information is also available on overseas hospices.

Institute of Family Therapy
24–32 Stephenson Way
London NW1 2HX
Tel: 020 7391 9150
Fax: 020 7391 9169
Email: ift@psyc.bbk.ac.uk
Offers counselling for families including those in which a family member has serious illness, disability or where there has been bereavement. Fees are on a self-assessed sliding scale.

Irish Cancer Society
43–45 Northumberland Road
Dublin 4
Republic of Ireland
Tel: 00353 (1)2310 500
Fax: 00353 (1) 2310 555
Email: info@irishcancer.ie
Website: www.cancer.ie
National Cancer Helpline:
Freefone 1800 200 700*
Email: Helpline@irishcancer.ie
Action Breast Cancer Helpline:
Freefone 1800 309 040*
Email: ABC@irishcancer.ie
National Smokers Quitline:
CallSave 1850 201 203*
Email: quitline@irishcancer.ie
*Please note that all the above numbers are accessible only from the Republic of Ireland.
    The Irish Cancer Society is Ireland's national cancer care charity, dedicated to eliminating cancer as a major health problem and improving the lives of those living with cancer through patient care, research and education.

Look Good . . . Feel Better

West Hill House
32 West Hill
Epsom
Surrey KT19 8JD
Tel: 01372 747 500
Fax: 01372 747 502
Email: info@lgfb.co.uk
Website: www.lookgoodfeelbetter.co.uk
The cancer support charity that helps women manage the visible side effects of cancer treatments.

You can download their brochure from the website or use the contact details above.

Lymphoedema Support Network

St Luke's Crypt
Sydney Street
London SW3 6NH
Office hours: 9.30 am–4.30 pm
Information and Support:
0207 351 4480
Administration: 0207 351 0990
Fax: 0207 349 9809
Email:
adminlsn@lymphoedema.freeserve.co.uk
Website: www.lymphoedema.org/lsn
The LSN provides information and support to people with lymphoedema. The charity produces a quarterly newsletter and wide range of factsheets. It works to raise awareness of lymphoedema and campaigns for better national standards of care.

Macmillan Cancer Support

89 Albert Embankment
London SE1 7UQ
Macmillan Cancer Support improves the lives of people affected by cancer. It provides practical, medical, emotional and financial support and campaigns for better cancer care. 'Cancer affects us all. We can all help.'

Macmillan CancerLine

Freephone: 0808 808 2020
Textphone: 0808 808 0121
(Mon–Fri, 9 am–9 pm)
Email: cancerline@macmillan.org.uk
Specialist advisers offer confidential advice and help you find the information you need.

Macmillan Benefits Advice Line

Freephone: 0800 500 800

South Asian lines (Freephone):

Hindi 0808 808 0100
Punjabi 0808 808 0101
Urdu 0808 808 0102
Open Mon–Fri, 9 am–6 pm

Macmillan YouthLine

Freephone: 0808 808 0800
(Mon–Fri, 9 am–9 pm)
Email: youthline@macmillan.org.uk
Are you between 12 and 21 years old? Are you affected by cancer? Do you need to talk to someone?

Maggie's
8 Newton Place
Glasgow G3 7PR
Tel: 0141 341 3343
Fax: 0141 341 5699
Email: media@maggiescentres.org
Website: www.maggiescentres,org
*Maggie's Centres are free, drop-in
information and support centres for
anybody who has, or who has had,
cancer. They are also for their families,
their friends and their carers. Each
centre is located on the grounds of a
major cancer hospital within short
walking distance of the oncology
department, and is open weekdays
from 9 am–5 pm.*

*Although physically close to the
hospital, walking into Maggie's is like
walking into a different world, with no
waiting rooms, no appointments, no
uniforms. Many people come in before,
after or between appointments, and
say even a short stop in Maggie's will
relieve the stress of a hospital visit.*

*Maggie's centres are known for their
remarkable approach, providing
support from cancer professionals in a
determinedly non-institutional
environment. People are invited into
the kitchen for a cup of tea and a chat
with one of the information and
support specialists, to browse the
library, see the benefits advisor or to
access one of the classes, for example,
T'ai Chi, yoga, relaxation, art therapy.*

Marie Curie Cancer Care
89 Albert Embankment
London SE1 7TP
Freephone: 0800 716 146
Tel: 020 7599 7777
Fax: 020 7599 7788
Email: info@mariecurie.org.uk
Website: www.mariecurie.org.uk
*Marie Curie Cancer Care provides
high-quality nursing totally free, to
give terminally ill people the choice of
dying at home, supported by their
families. Marie Curie Nurses provide
practical, hands-on care, and will
typically spend a full shift with their
patient, often overnight. Marie Curie
Nursing is arranged through the
patient's district nurse or GP.*

*The charity also runs 10 Marie
Curie Hospices, which actively
promote quality of life for people with
cancer and provide support for their
families. Hospices are located in
Belfast, Caterham (Surrey), North
London, Solihull, Penarth (near
Cardiff), Liverpool, Bradford,
Newcastle, Glasgow and Edinburgh.
There is also a Marie Curie day
therapy unit in Tiverton, Devon.*

Medicines and Healthcare Regulatory Agency (MHRA)
10-2 Market Towers
1 Nine Elms Lane
London SW8 5NQ
Tel: 020 7084 2000
(Mon–Fri, 9 am–5 pm)
020 7210 3000 (all other times)
Fax: 020 7084 2353
Email: info@mhra.gsi.gov.uk
Contact the MHRA for the booklet on safety of breast implants referred to in Chapter 3.

The Patients Association
PO Box 935
Harrow
Middlesex HA1 3YJ
Helpline: 0845 608 4455
(020 8423 8999 for local callers)
Office only: 020 8423 9111
Email: mailbox@patients-association.com
The Patients Association is an independent national charity providing patients with an opportunity to raise concerns and share experiences of healthcare.

Through the Helpline, correspondence and research, the association learns from patients the issues that are of concern and works towards improving healthcare for all.

Tak Tent Cancer Support Scotland
Flat 530 Shelley Court
Gartnavel Complex
Glasgow G12 0YN
Helpline: 0141 211 0122
Offers information and support for cancer patients, families, friends and associated professionals. Provides a network of support groups in West and Central Scotland including young adult group (16–25 years). Counselling and complementary therapy services are available.

Tenovus Cancer Information Centre
Velindre Hospital
Velindre Road
Whitchurch
Cardiff CF14 2TL
Cancer Helpline:
Freephone 0808 808 1010
Tel: 0292 019 6100
Fax: 0192 019 6105
Email: tcic1@velindre-tr.wales.nhs.uk
Website: www.tenovus.com
Provides information and advice on all cancer-related concerns. Contact via the Helpline, by letter or personal visit.

Tourism For All
Shap Road Industrial Estate
Shap Road
Kendal
Cumbria LA9 6NZ
Tel: 0845 124 9973 (direct line)
Tel: 0845 345 1970 (general
enquiries)
*Advice and information on holidays
and travel arrangements for people
who are disabled or elderly.*

Ulster Cancer Foundation
40–44 Eglantine Avenue
Belfast BT9 6DX
Helpline: Freephone 0800 783 3339
Tel: 028 9066 3281
Fax: 028 9066 8715
Email: infocis@ulstercancer.org
*A cancer information and helpline
service. Also provides support services
such as counselling, art therapy and
support groups throughout the
province, and volunteer befriender
visits. Breast cancer fitting service for
supply of specialist bras and
swimwear. Services are provided
throughout Northern Ireland.*

Women's Health Concern
Whitehall House
41 Whitehall
London SW1A 2BY
Tel: 0845 123 2319
(Mon–Tue, 10 am–2 pm,
Wed–Fri, 10 am–1 pm)
Fax: 020 7925 1505
Email: counselling@womens-health-
concern.org
Website: www.womens-health-concern.org
*Women's Health Concern is the UK's
leading charity providing help and
advice to women on a wide variety of
gynaecological and sexual health
conditions. Unbiased, accurate
information helps women understand
more about their problem, allowing
them to feel confident about discussing
the diagnostic process and treatment
options with their doctor. Women can
speak directly with nurses or email
their query to Women's Health
Concern (all emails are answered
within 48 hours). They can also
download information from the
website about gynaecological and
sexual health problems.*

Complementary care

**British Holistic
Medical Association**
BHMA Administrator
PO Box 371
Bridgwater
Somerset
TA6 9BG
Tel: 01278 722000
Email: admin@bhma.org
Website: www.bmha.org
*Aims to educate doctors and other
healthcare professionals so that
patients are treated as individuals.
Publishes a quarterly magazine,
Holistic Health, for members, also
self-help cassettes and books. Holds
annual conferences. Send SAE for
information.*

**Institute for
Complementary Medicine**
Unit 25
Tavern Quay Business Centre
Sweden Gate
London SE16 7TX
Tel: 020 7231 5855
Fax: 020 7237 5175
Email: info@i-c-m.org.uk
Website: www.i-c-m.org.uk
*Facilitates the British Register of
Complementary Practitioners and can
supply names of highly qualified
practitioners of various kinds of
complementary medicine, such as
homeopathy, reflexology,
aromatherapy, massage and*

*relaxation. Also has contact with
other support groups. Please send SAE
and two first class stamps for
information, stating area of interest.*

New Approaches to Cancer
PO Box 194
Chertsey
Surrey KT16 0WJ
Tel: 0800 389 2662
Email: help@anac.org.uk
Website: www.anac.org.uk
*New Approaches to Cancer is an
organisation started by a group of four
colleagues, two doctors and two
healers, in 1969. They felt it was
important to share with as many
people as possible the positive
experience of using 'Gentle Therapies'
and that these, combined with
supportive counselling, self-help
groups and dietary advice could make a
real difference to people going through
the experience of cancer. New
Approaches to Cancer provides a
nationwide information service that is
easily accessible and free to all. Over
the past year the charity has extended
and improved its services, and will
continue to offer the care, attention,
love and education that the charity is
so well known for.*

*All services are free of charge. The
charity provides a wide range of
information on experienced holistic
practitioners and clinics nationwide
and runs self-help groups in Surrey,
Sussex and Middlesex. It organises*

talks and healthy living demonstrations, runs regular classes in holistic therapy to support cancer patients such as relaxation and visualisation, yoga, nutrition, flower remedies, life coaching, etc. In the spirit of prevention, it invites local medical practitioners and nurses to attend as well as patients' families and friends.

Penny Brohn Cancer Care
Chapel Pill Lane
Pill
Bristol BS20 0HH
Helpline: 0845 123 23 10
Tel: 01275 370 100
Fax: 01275 370 101
Email: helpline@pennybrohn.org
Website: www.pennybrohncancercare.org
Penny Brohn Cancer Care provides complementary care to people with cancer and their loved ones. It offers practical self-help techniques to improve quality of life and to help manage the fear of cancer. Will usually involve some cost.

Acupuncture

British Acupuncture Council
63 Jeddo Road
London W12 9HQ
Tel: 020 8735 0400
Fax: 020 8735 0404
Email: info@acupuncture.org.uk
Website: www.acupuncture.org.uk
The British Acupuncture Council is the largest registering body for professional acupuncturists in the UK, with over 2800 members. Its aim is to ensure the health and safety of the public at all times whilst maintaining high standards of education, ethics, discipline and practice among its members. All members have undertaken a minimum of three years' training in acupuncture and biomedical sciences appropriate to the practice of acupuncture. They carry the letters MBAcC after their name. It is committed to funding research and increasing the role that traditional acupuncture plays in the health and well-being of the nation.

A copy of the full Register of Practitioner Members can be obtained by sending a cheque for £5 to the address above. Alternatively, a list of practitioners in your area can be requested free of charge. Simply telephone, email, fax or write.

British Medical Acupuncture Society
Royal London Homoeopathic
Hospital
60 Great Ormond Street
London WC1N 3HR
Email: Admin@medical-acupuncture.org.uk
Website: www.medical-acupuncture.co.uk
Promotes the use and understanding of acupuncture as part of the practice of medicine. Trains qualified doctors and other regulated health professionals. Publishes a journal. A patient information leaflet and details of practitioners are available on request.

Art therapy

British Association of Art Therapists Ltd
24–27 White Lion Street
London N1 9PD
Tel: 020 7686 4216
Fax: 020 7837 7945
Email: info@baat.org
Website: www.baat.org
The British Association of Art Therapists provides information about art therapy (free of charge) and runs regular courses and events.

Person-centred Art Therapy Association
Belinda Mcleod
Aubrich House
17 Kelvin Brook
Hurst Park, West Plesey
Surrey KT8 1RT
Person-centred Art Therapy Association is for those holding a certificate in Person-centred Art Therapy Skills to meet, share theory and practice.

Counselling

British Association for Counselling and Psychotherapy
BACP House
15 St John's Business Park
Lutterworth
Leicestershire LE17 4HB
Tel: 0870 443 5166
Fax: 0870 443 5161
Email: bacp@bacp.co.uk
Website: www.bacp.co.uk
BACP has an online directory of therapists which can be accessed from the Find a Therapist button on the website home page. The same information, in hard copy, can be requested from the BACP Information Office. Useful information about choosing a therapist is available from both sources.

Healing

**Confederation
of Healing Organisations**
Tel: 01584 890662 (Administrator)
Email: Diane.Schooley@btinternet.com
*The Confederation of Healing
Organisations provides contact and
distant healing from its member
associations with around 4000
healers in the UK. All are regulated by
the same compulsory Code and
Disciplinary Procedures, covered by
public liability and professional
indemnity insurance comparable to a
GP's and accept the same minimum
criteria for entry and training. No
belief is required of patients. Fees, if
any, are moderate. The DH has advised
that their Patient's Charter entitles
patients wishing to see a healer to
request this in NHS hospitals.*

**National Federation of Spiritual
Healers (NFSH)**
Old Manor Farm Studio
Church Street
Sunbury-on-Thames
Middlesex TW16 6RG
Referrals only: 0891 616 080
Tel: 0845 123 2777
Fax: 0193 277 9648
Email: office@nfsh.org.uk
Website: www.nfsh.org.uk
*The object of the NFSH is to serve the
public good by the promotion of the
study and practice of the art and
science of spiritual healing. NFSH*
*maintains a list of member healers in
all parts of the UK. Healers are allowed
to visit and treat patients in NHS
hospitals by invitation of the patients.*

Herbalism

**National Institute
of Medical Herbalists**
Elm House
54 Mary Arches Street
Exeter
Devon EX4 3BA
Telephone: 01392 426022
Fax: 01392 498963
Email: admin@nimh.org.uk
Website: www.nimh.org.uk
*The oldest professional body for
medical herbalists. All members have a
minimum of three years' training in
medicine. Maintains a strict Ethical
Code and accredits degree courses.
Write, telephone or email enquiries for
a registered practitioner in your area
and for information on herbal
medicine.*

**College of Practitioners
of Phytotherapy**
Oak Glade
9 Hythe Close
Polegate
East Sussex BN26 6LQ
Tel: 01323 484353
Email: pamela.bull@btopenworld.com
*Provides a register of qualified
herbalists in the UK and elsewhere.*

Homeopathy

British Homeopathic Association
Hahnemann House
29 Park Street West
Luton LU1 3BE
Tel: 0870 444 3950
Website: www.trusthomeopathy.org
The BHA provides a list of medically-qualified doctors who practise homeopathy working in hospitals, as GPs or in private practice, throughout the UK and overseas. A free information pack is available and includes information on how to get homeopathy on the NHS and a copy of our bi-monthly magazine Health and Homeopathy.

Society of Homoeopaths
11 Brookfield
Duncan Close
Moulton Park
Northampton NN3 6WL
Tel: 0845 450 6611
Email: info@homeopathy-soh.org
Website: www.homeopathy-soh.org
Society of Homeopaths is the largest organisation representing professional homeopaths in Europe with over 1500 members on its register.
Visit the website to find your local practitioner and to find out more information about homeopathy.

Massage: aromatherapy

International Federation of Aromatherapists
61–63 Churchfield Road
London W3 6AY
Tel: 020 8992 8945
Fax: 020 8992 7983
Website: www.ifaroma.org
For written enquiries, please send SAE.

The International Federation of Professional Aromatherapists (IFPA)
IFPA House
82 Ashby Road
Hinckley
Leicestershire LE10 1SN
Tel: 01455 637987
Fax: 01455 890956
Email: admin@ifparoma.org
Website: www.ifparoma.org
IFPA is a rapidly expanding professional aromatherapy federation with truly international membership. It offers professional credibility, a quarterly journal and many other benefits to its members. Please contact the office for a list of practitioners within your local area.

Massage: reflexology

Association of Reflexologists
5 Fore Street
Taunton
TA1 1HX
Tel: 0870 567 3320
Email: info@aor.org.uk
Website: www.aor.org.uk
*Membership organisation for
reflexology practitioners providing
membership services including
insurance. Awarding body for
reflexology schools following set
curriculum and training to published
standards. Publishes quarterly
reflexology journal,* Reflexions. *Full
members denoted by the initials MAR.*

British Reflexology Association
Monks Orchard
Whitbourne
Worcester WR6 5RB
Tel: 01886 821207
Fax: 01886 822017
Email: bra@britreflex.co.uk
Website: www.britreflex.co.uk
*The British Reflexology Association
was founded in 1985 to act as a
representative body for persons
practising the method of Reflexology
as a profession and for students
training in the method. The BRA
publishes a* Register of Members
(£3.00) and a quarterly newsletter,
Footprints. *The official teaching body
for the BRA is The Bayly School of
Reflexology. A register of members is*

*available and details of reflexology
training courses, books and charts can
be supplied.*

Naturopathy

**General Council and Register
of Naturopaths**
2 Goswell Road
Street
Somerset BA16 0JG
Tel: 01458 840072
Fax: 01458 840075
Email: admin@naturopathy.org.uk
Website: www.naturopathy.org.uk
*The General Council and Register of
Naturopaths is the largest
naturopathic register in the UK. It sets
and monitors educational standards in
naturopathic training, sets and
enforces a Code of Ethics, and
publishes annually a list of suitably
qualified naturopathic practitioners,
for the benefit and protection of the
public. The GCRN operates, in
association with the British
Naturopathic Association, a
HealthLine service for the public,
which can be contacted using the
details above.*

Traditional Chinese Medicine

Association of Traditional Chinese Medicine (ATCM)
1 Cline Road
London N11 2LY
Tel: 020 8361 2121
Fax: 020 8361 2121
Email: info@atcm.co.uk
Main regulatory body in the UK. Maintains a register of 700 professionally qualified TCM practitioners.

Yoga

British Wheel of Yoga
25 Jermyn Street
Sleaford
Lincolnshire
NG34 7RU
Tel: 01529 306 851
Fax: 01529 303 233
Email: office@bwy.org.uk
Website: www.bwy.org.uk
Encouragement and help for people to understand all aspects of yoga and its practice; maintains standards of yoga teaching, organises and supports local branches. Publications list available.

Index

Have you found *Breast Cancer: Answers at your fingertips* useful and practical? If so, you may be interested in other books from Class Publishing.

BREAST RECONSTRUCTION:
YOUR CHOICE £19.99

Dick Rainsbury and Virginia Straker

Every week, hundreds of women are faced with a diagnosis of breast cancer. At such a difficult time, they need information, answers and support in making the best choices for them.

This practical guide is based around the experiences of more than 60 women who have lived through this emotional helter-skelter. It explains all the available surgical and non-surgical options, and covers all you need to know to help you make your decision about breast reconstruction. It will give you that extra confidence you need.

TYPE 1 DIABETES:
Answers at your fingertips £14.99
TYPE 2 DIABETES:
Answers at your fingertips £14.99

Dr Charles Fox and Dr Anne Kilvert

The latest edition of our bestselling reference guide on diabetes has now been split into two books covering the two distinct forms of the disease. These books maintain the popular question and answer format to provide practical advice for patients on every aspect of living with the condition.

'I have no hesitation in commending this book.'

Sir Steve Redgrave CBE,
Vice President, Diabetes UK

DUMP YOUR TOXIC WAIST! £14.99

Dr Derrick Cutting

The easy, drug-free and medically accurate way to lose inches, beat diabetes and stop that heart attack.

'. . . an excellent book for those who are interested in unclogging their arteries, or getting down to their ideal weight for good, or controlling their blood pressure, or discovering a new vitality'

The Family Heart Digest

MIGRAINE:
Answers at your fingertips £14.99

Dr Manuela Fontebasso

Written by an experienced GP with a special interest in headache and migraine, this book acknowledges the uniqueness of every sufferer's experience. Communication between patient and professional is crucial if this complex condition is to be addressed and the best treatment prescribed.

This book will help you understand the nature of your headache, and give you the confidence to be involved in all areas of decision making.

MENOPAUSE:
Answers at your fingertips £17.99

Dr Heather Currie

The average age of the menopause is 51 years, but it can occur much earlier or later. The symptoms vary widely in their severity, and can include hot flushes, night sweats, palpitations, insomnia, joint pain and headaches. Women are at greater risk of osteoporosis after the menopause.

This invaluable guide answers hundreds of questions from women approaching or experiencing the menopause, and provides positive, practical advice on a range of issues.

BEATING DEPRESSION £17.99

Dr Stefan Cembrowicz
and Dr Dorcas Kingham

Depression is one of most common illnesses in the world – affecting up to one in four people at some time in their lives. This book shows sufferers and their families that they are not alone, and offers tried and tested techniques for overcoming depression.

'All you need to know about depression, presented in a clear, concise and readable way.'

Ann Dawson
World Health Organization

PRIORITY ORDER FORM

Cut out or photocopy this form and send it (post free in the UK) to:

Class Publishing   **Tel: 01256 302 699**
FREEPOST 16705   **Fax: 01256 812 558**
Macmillan Distribution
Basingstoke RG21 6ZZ

Please send me urgently   *Post included*
(tick below)   *price per copy (UK only)*

☐ **Breast Cancer: Answers at your fingertips** (ISBN 978 1 85959 198 7)   £17.99

☐ **Breast Reconstruction: Your Choices** (ISBN 978 1 85959 197 0)   £22.99

☐ **Type 1 Diabetes: Answers at your fingertips** (ISBN 978 1 85959 175 8)   £17.99

☐ **Type 2 Diabetes: Answers at your fingertips** (ISBN 978 1 85959 176 5)   £17.99

☐ **Migraine: Answers at your fingertips** (ISBN 978 1 85959 170 3)   £17.99

☐ **Menopause: Answers at your fingertips** (ISBN 978 1 85959 155 0)   £20.99

☐ **Dump Your Toxic Waist!** (ISBN 978 1 85959 191 8)   £17.99

☐ **Beating Depression** (ISBN 978 1 85959 150 5)   £20.99

TOTAL _____

Easy ways to pay

Cheque: I enclose a cheque payable to Class Publishing for £ _____

Credit card: Please debit my   Mastercard   ☐ Visa   ☐ Amex   ☐ Switch

Number _____   Expiry date _____

Name _____

My address for delivery is _____

_____

Town _____ County _____ Postcode _____

Telephone number (*in case of query*) _____

Credit card billing address if different from above _____

_____

Town _____ County _____ Postcode _____

Class Publishing's guarantee: remember that if, for any reason, you are not satisfied with these books, we will refund all your money, without any questions asked. Prices and VAT rates may be altered for reasons beyond our control.